Physical Therapy Management

Physical Therapy Management

Ron Scott, PT, JD, EdD, LLM, MSBA
Attorney-Mediator and Clinical Physical Therapist/Educator
Cibolo, Texas

Christopher Petrosino, PT, PhD
Director/Associate Professor
Krannert School of Physical Therapy
University of Indianapolis
Indianapolis, Indiana

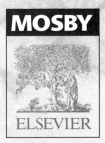

MOSBY

ELSEVIER

CONTRIBUTOR

Jonathan Cooperman, PT, DPT, MS, JD
President, Ohio Physical Therapy Association;
Supervisor, Akron General Medical Center
Health and Wellness Center,
North Stow, Ohio

MOSBY
ELSEVIER

11830 Westline Industrial Drive
St. Louis, Missouri 63146

Notice

Neither the Publisher nor the Editors/Authors assume any responsibility for any loss or injury and/or damage to persons or property arising out of or related to any use of the material contained in this book. It is the responsibility of the treating practitioner, relying on independent expertise and knowledge of the patient, to determine the best treatment and method of application for the patient.

The Publisher

Library of Congress Control Number 2007920576

Publishing Director: Linda Duncan
Senior Editor: Kathy Falk
Developmental Editor: Megan Fennell
Publishing Services Manager: Pat Joiner-Myers
Senior Project Manager: David Stein
Design Manager: Andrea Lutes

Printed in the United States

Last digit is the print number: 9 8 7 6 5 4 3 2 1

The authors dedicate this work to all the past, current, and future physical therapy managers who have made, make, and will make this dynamic vital system all that it must be to serve patients, their significant others, and society.

Ron Scott also dedicates his contribution to his wife of 34 years, Pepi, for her tireless belief in him, and for her dedication and support throughout the years they have been together.

Chris Petrosino also dedicates his work to his wife, Rebecca, and their two sons, Adam and Stephen.

Jonathan Cooperman also dedicates his chapter to his wife, Tracey.

Preface

Health care clinical management is one of the most complex yet rewarding professional endeavors that can be undertaken. Physical therapy clinical management (most often carried out by physical therapists) involves the masterful execution of a myriad of important functions. These include, among many other coprimary objectives, selection of a business site; the establishment of a clinical mission and goals; the recruitment, selection, and retention of key human resources; the everyday management of patient care services; and patient, client, and relevant third-party satisfaction. Physical therapy clinical services managers must also be (and must ensure that their staffs are) on the cutting edge of legal, regulatory, and ethical compliance at multiple tiered levels—from federal to state to local governmental mandates to directives of accreditation entities and professional associations.

Managed care has fundamentally changed the rules of engagement and operations for physical therapy clinical services managers. For the first time in medical history, cost containment is a coprimary objective of health care delivery, along with optimal patient care service delivery. Although managed care makes a clinical manager's job more complex, it does not make it unreasonably more difficult.

Managed care is not a bad phenomenon. The health care delivery system costs society an increasing percentage of the gross national product every year. It is the duty of clinical health care services directors to be good and responsible stewards of their budgets and of health care expenditures at multiple levels.

Managed care has not, however, fundamentally altered the legal and professional ethical duties of clinical health services managers and their professional and support staffs. They are still and always fiduciaries toward patients and clients under their care. As fiduciaries, they are charged by law to place patients' and clients' interests above all others, including their own.

Physical therapy clinical services managers have traditionally done a stellar job of multitasking and managing these roles. Rather than recommending wholesale reconfiguration of their skills bag, this book's premise is that they are already there.

The book is written for future (professional and postprofessional students) and for current physical therapy clinical services managers. It contains a wide array of cases, exercises, and questions designed to stimulate higher-order thinking and perhaps debate. Chapter 1, "Dynamic Nature of Management in Health Care Organizations," showcases the health care organization. The chapter details its attributes: organizational behavior, culture, forms, and structures. Chapter 2, "Human Resource Management in Physical Therapy Settings," addresses human resource or people management. It has been said that human resource management is as critically important to patient life and death as is the rendition of health care services. Chapter 3, "Physical Therapy Reimbursement and Financial Management," presents facts and issues surrounding health care finance and marketing or services. Chapter 4, "Legal and Ethical Management Issues," written by Jonathan Cooperman, focuses on legal and professional ethical problems, issues, and dilemmas. The book concludes with Chapter 5, "Information, Quality, and Risk Management." Much of this chapter focuses on management responsibilities associated with the Health Insurance Portability and Accountability Act (HIPAA). You will hopefully be pleasantly surprised to learn that HIPAA compliance is not as onerous as it is rumored to be.

Best wishes for continuing practice and management success!

Contents

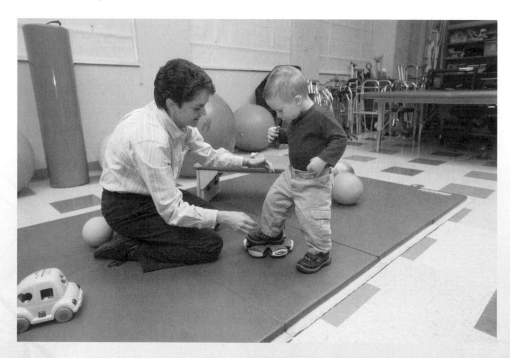

Courtesy University of Indianapolis.

CHAPTER 1

Dynamic Nature of Management in Health Care Organizations

Christopher Petrosino

ABSTRACT

Physical therapists frequently move into management positions without the knowledge, skill, or decision-making abilities that are needed to optimize the potential for success of the department or clinic. Although the learning curve is steep, many therapists succeed as a result of determination, perseverance, and the inherent attributes required in patient/client management. To help future managers better negotiate the learning curve, this chapter provides them with a foundation from which to develop the knowledge of health care organizational behavior, design, and theory; the skills of managing people and becoming a leader; and the ability to drive an organization through strategic planning and critical decision making.

KEY WORDS AND PHRASES

Accommodation
Arbitration
Avoiding
Bureaucracy
Centralization
Change
Coaching
Collaboration
Communication
Competition
Compromise
Contingency theory
Decentralized

Decision making
Delegating
Differentiation
Directive
Director
Formative evaluation
Goals
Integration
Leader
Macroenvironmental
Management
Managers
Mediation

Microenvironment
Mission statement
Objectives
Organizational design
Organizational structure
Power
Strategic planning
Summative evaluation
Supporting
Values
Vision statement

1. Understand business organizations as social microsystems that develop structure from varying levels of bureaucracy.

2. Develop and adapt organizational policies to meet the needs and desires of both the organization and the individuals within it.

3. Compare and contrast the two principal types of business organizations: closed and open.

4. Apply appropriate leadership in a crisis situation.

5. Ascertain the position of individual employees according to the hierarchy of need fulfillment, and determine how best to help them achieve self-actualization.

6. Effectively negotiate or mediate issues for successful problem resolution, including organizational changes, with employees and relevant others.

7. Teach employees in physical therapy clinical settings about basic negotiation principles.

ORGANIZATIONAL DESIGN AND THEORY

Organizational design is the way people consciously coordinate, develop, and modify the structure of an organization to optimize function. A successful design depends on the ability of those in leadership positions to organize and manage people toward the achievement of **goals**. The roots of organizational design arguably date to the ancient Egyptians, the Far East dynasties, or the Mayan civilization. One could imagine the highly structured system of organization needed to develop such social networks, cultural complexities, and architectural accomplishments. There must have been coordination and control from someone in authority who established **communication** channels, assigned work, and structured procedures. Although the organizational design and structure of our ancient civilizations inform modern organization, they have not received as much acclaim for the impact on organizational design as has the Industrial Revolution of the late 1700s and 1800s.

The science of modern **management** started on two fronts, one in America and the other in Europe, yet both focused on managing workers for the effective accomplishment of goals. Henry R. Towne (1844-1924), an American engineer with management savvy, initiated the science of management by proposing five stages to manage work: (1) gaining knowledge of machines and human work, (2) using the knowledge to formulate applicable laws and formulas, (3) using science to establish optimal performance standards for machines and humans, (4) reorganizing processes from the findings, and (5) establishing cooperation between labor and management. Following Towne's lead, Frederick W. Taylor (1856-1915), also known as the "Father of Scientific Management," developed four principles of scientific management: (1) replacement of old methods with a true science of managing, with laws, rules, and principles; (2) selection, training, and development of workers on the basis of scientific principles; (3) emphasis on cooperation of **managers** and workers for compliance with scientific principles; and (4) division of tasks and responsibilities among workers and managers. Taylor and his associates believed that each person should have clearly defined daily tasks with the resources and environmental conditions to accomplish the task. When the worker completed the task, higher pay was given. Less pay was given to those who did not complete their task. As an organization grows, some tasks can be completed only by workers with a certain expertise, thus initiating a division of labor based on qualifications. In Europe, a French mining engineer named Henri Fayol (1841-1925) concentrated on applying a scientific approach to upper administration and earned the title of "Father of Modern Management." In consideration of administrative responsibilities, Fayol stressed the importance of planning for the future, organization of people and resources, compliance of workers, coordination of activities, and adherence to rules. He identified the 14 principles of management found in Box 1-1.

As Towne, Taylor, and Fayol focused on recommendations for the operation of organizations, Max Weber (1864-1920) focused on **organizational structure** with an emphasis on division of labor with specialization, authority hierarchy, appropriate selection of workers with a career orientation, and adherence to rules and regulations. Unfortunately, Weberian **bureaucracy** has become tinged with association to rule-encumbered inefficiency and impersonal authoritarian managers.

BOX **1-1** ■ **Fayol's 14 Principles of Management**

1. Workers are divided into groups to permit specialization (Division of Labor).
2. Authority should equal the responsibilities of the position held (Authority).
3. Discipline is required for task completion, motivation, and respect (Discipline).
4. Workers should report to only one superior (Unity of Command).
5. There should be one manager and one plan for operations with the same objective (Unity of Direction).
6. Organization interests take precedence over individual or group interests (Subordination of Individual Interests to General Interests).
7. Rewards for work should be fair (Remuneration).
8. Each initiative or task should have appropriate degree of centralization or decentralization (Centralization).
9. There should be a clear line of authority (Scalar Chain).
10. Keep the workplace, the work, and the worker in order (Order).
11. Treat workers with kindness and justice (Equity).
12. Minimize worker turnover to ensure goal accomplishment (Stability of Tenure Personnel).
13. Allow workers to develop through freedom of creation and execution of plans (Initiative).
14. Encourage harmony, rapport building, and union among workers (Esprit de Corps).

Nonetheless, a clear definition of authority and responsibility, through division of labor among qualified workers, increases efficiency. For example, appropriate division of labor among physical therapists, physical therapist assistants, and physical therapist aides will most likely improve efficiency. Maintaining the authority hierarchy and following the formal rules set by the organization, accrediting agencies, and government alleviate some concern for arbitrary and capricious actions, personal subjugation, nepotism, and potentially ill-informed subjective judgments. Bureaucracy is an efficient means of organizing and continues to be a central feature in modern organizations. Likewise, care must be taken not to fall into bureaucratic rigidity, in which a rule is blindly followed without appreciation of the intent or misused as an end in itself to control workers. Furthermore, workers must not "work to the rules," a tendency that creates a minimal level of acceptable performance and does not allow the organization to move forward.

Bureaucratic structures vary in complexity and may range from a very simple structure with little support staff, division of labor, and a small administrative hierarchy to a Weberian structure of a mechanistic bureaucracy with considerable formalization and a high degree of centralized authority to a loosely structured, highly specialized professional bureaucracy. Physical therapy clinical practices, like all business organizations, operate along a continuum from the closed, mechanistic, internally focused, "slow," reactive bureaucracy at one end of the spectrum to the open, organic, fluid, and proactive business organization at the other. No organization is wholly "closed" or "open," and while it may seem that the aforementioned traits ascribed to a bureaucracy are inherently undesirable, that is not always true. One might assume that most physical therapy practices are organized as an "open" professional bureaucracy wherein a relatively decentralized administration relies on the highly specialized skills and knowledge of the physical therapist to function effectively. In this scenario, a professional is hired and given considerable control over accomplishment of duties within the constraints of a set of standards. However, physical therapy practices exist along an ever-changing continuum of open to closed structure. Some health care organizations are moving toward a closed structure in search of some control over the challenges to maintain or gain a share of the health care market. Max Weber first described the classic closed, bureaucratic organization in 1920.

In contrast to the closed organization, the open, organic organization exists at the opposite end of the spectrum (Box 1-2). The open business organization is receiving attention as the emerging gold standard among health care organizations in the managed care era. Its focus on professional employee empowerment, independence and creativity, and proactive management of crises from reimbursement to scope of practice issues makes its prevalence promising for organizational survival. Yet without adherence to clearly defined policy and procedures, an open organization can leave workers less constrained and more defiant of administrative authority. Therefore each organization must adhere to a structure that best accomplishes the organization's vision, mission, and goals, which

---

BOX **1-2** ■ **Comparison of Characteristics of Closed- (Versus Open-) Structure Organizations**

Characteristics of a Closed-Structure Organization	Characteristics of an Open-Structure Organization
Heavily laden with rules and regulations	Eschews the existence of, and/or adherence to, rigid organizational rules and regulations
Rigid and detailed documentation standards	
Standardization of processes	Individual autonomy and creativity critically important to operational success
Strict division of labor, based on worker expertise	
Highly centralized decision making	Multi-skilling and cross-training common
Clear, formal chain of command, as evidenced by a wire-diagrammed organizational chart	Decision making decentralized to operational work groups
Employee advancement exclusively on the basis of merit	Relative unimportance of formal chain of command within the organization
A sense of depersonalization of the individual; interpersonal orientation expressly designed to prevent favoritism, promote uniformity, and ensure equity	Less career orientation among employees than in a bureaucracy
	Key characteristics of the organization: job satisfaction and adaptability
Operations typically led by professional managers, not by the business owners	
Primarily internally focused, without substantial regard for the external environment; hence the label "closed organization"	

---

typically results in some balance on a continuum between bureaucratic and open-systems design.

According to Hage's axiomatic theory, the organizational means (structural input variables) and ends (behavioral outputs) of bureaucracies and open systems are at polar opposites. The following grid summarizes Hage's model.

Organizational Means (Inputs)		
	Bureaucracy	**Open System**
Formalization	High	Low
Centralization	High	Low
Stratification	High	Low
Complexity	Low	High

Organizational Ends (Outputs)		
	Bureaucracy	**Open System**
Efficiency	High	Low
Productivity	High	Low
Job satisfaction	Low	High
Adaptability	Low	High

EXERCISE **1-1**

Discuss in small groups whether you agree with Hage's model for classification of bureaucracies and open organizations. Why or why not? Share results with the larger group.

According to Hage's axiomatic theory, the more bureaucratic an organization becomes, the higher the efficiency and productivity, whereas the more open the organization becomes, the greater potential for employees to be satisfied about their work and for the company to adapt quickly to a changing market. Caution must be taken when making business decisions on the basis of generalizations, and all constraints affecting the organization must be considered when adopting any variation on organizational design.

Whether "open" or "closed," each organizational type has inherent advantages and disadvantages over the other, and variations on the continuum have developed with emphasis on refining either the means of organizational efficiency or the ends of obtaining desired outcomes.

Through the propagation of management science during the industrial revolution, other management designs and strategies have developed focusing on different aspects of efficiency and outcome. Administrators and researchers have focused on the function of interdependent and interrelated parts, motivation and leadership, situational influences and strategies, continuous improvement in processes and quality, and various management styles.

Organizational Structure

Organizational structure is the degree to which an organization enacts formal or informal rules of behavior, centralized or decentralized control of operations, **differentiation** or **integration** of work, and the complexity of relationships among employees.

Formal and informal rules of behavior are well defined in bureaucratic organizations. The level of formalization in a physical therapy practice can easily be assessed through observation of superior/subordinate interaction and review of the department's policy and procedures manual and job descriptions. The degree to which the written documents of the practice describe the rights and duties of the physical therapist, physical therapist assistant, department aide or technician, and other staff members (e.g., receptionists, billing clerks, clerical workers), as well as how those rights and duties are handled by employees, constitutes the level of formalization in the practice. The level of formalization gives authority to those who hold superior positions within the organization, such as a physical therapy manager over a staff physical therapist. An organizational chart provides a visual depiction of superior/subordinate positions within the organization; however, the chart may not be the best way of determining individuals responsible for making operation and planning decisions.

All physical therapy practices have a hierarchy of authority with which to make decisions. **Centralization** is a term used to describe the degree to which the top administrator has control over **decision making** for planning and operations. A highly centralized organization is sometimes referred to as a *top-down administration*, in which upper administrators make decisions and delegate responsibilities to subordinates. In a **decentralized** business, employees are divided into operating units in which a team **leader** or unit manager is responsible for planning and controlling operations. For instance, in larger hospitals a physical therapist may be designated the orthopedic team leader or the manager of industrial physical therapy and given specific supervision, operations, and planning responsibilities; this person is accountable to the department **director**.

The degree to which there is differentiation or integration of work depends on the specialized knowledge needed to perform the essential function of a job. More complex tasks may require a greater specialization of knowledge and skill to adequately complete the tasks. Occupational specialties require those responsible for completing the complex tasks to have specific qualifications and competencies, such as being licensed as a physical therapist or physical therapist assistant. This differentiation by qualifications results in what Max Weber termed "division of labor." Ideally, the division of labor leads to greater efficiency in production and outcomes. Nonetheless, efficiency may also be improved by integration of general tasks into the duties of those who are identified as having the time and capabilities to accomplish the less specialized task. One type of integration of duties used in health care is referred to as *cross-training*. More prevalent in rehabilitation facilities, home health agencies, and services for children, cross-training can enable a physical therapist or other health professional to screen patients in need of referral to another discipline or provide an adequate level of care to meet patient needs without multiple disciplines involvement. However, conflict can arise when scope of practice issues are breached or cross-training encroaches upon the specialized knowledge viewed as unique to a specific discipline. For instance, a physical therapist fabricating a splint could anger an occupational therapist; conversely, an occupational therapist evaluating gait could anger a physical therapist. Such a reaction may occur regardless of the competence of the individual performing the task. Within a physical therapy practice, differentiation and integration of duties should be regulated through a degree of formalization.

The complexity of relationships among superiors and subordinates has a profound impact on productivity, efficiency, and job satisfaction. A bureaucratic organization features an impersonal orientation to interpersonal relationships within the organization. Decisions are perceived as having a basis in well-defined roles, policies, procedures, and rules and regulations. Although informal lines of communication (often referred to as "the grapevine") do have a significant impact on relationships and outcomes, more formal lines of communication minimize anarchy. In a more bureaucratic organization, a higher **power** differential exists and results in relationships in which those in authority are expected to delegate tasks and those who are subordinates are expected to follow the direction of a supervisor. A more open system has fewer constraints on relationships and a lesser power differential. With a lesser power differential, there may be a greater degree of **collaboration** among superiors and subordinates in decision making, which can either create a more collegial atmosphere with greater autonomy or produce more conflict through subordinates challenging the authority of superiors.

Consider the relative advantages and disadvantages of open and closed designs in relation to organizational structure and the need for appropriate individualized balance within an organization. Formalization within a physical therapy practice could either improve efficiency or create administrative red tape. The classic bureaucracy is criticized for its relative unresponsiveness to **change** (especially rapid change). While strict organizational rules and regulations result in clear standards for official conduct, uniformity of application, and relative stability, such rigidity may lead to individual and collective goal displacement. It is not uncommon to hear physical therapists complain about the amount of time required for documentation or meetings that take away time from patient care. Likewise, the specialization and division of labor produce experts in focused fields, which is of great importance in clinical physical therapy. However, specialization may lead to diminished general competence and boredom. Formalization and specialization can result in a career orientation, which can be a strong incentive for employee loyalty to the organization. However, a career orientation does not inherently enhance productivity. The impersonal orientation of a bureaucracy can reduce the complexity of relationships and foster equitable treatment of all workers, but there is also the risk of creating a sterile environment with low morale. Power struggles may still develop therein. The centralized hierarchy of organizational authority maximizes coordination within the organization but often has the incidental disadvantage of decreased communication. Decreased communication typically results when employees do not view superiors as accessible, approachable, or responsive to concerns. Also, the importance of informal communication networks may be short-changed. A decentralized decision-making structure may result in better decisions because managers are closer to the operations, can anticipate and react quickly, and the structure builds the leadership skills of employees. However, decentralizing decision-making authority can negatively affect the practice because managers or team leaders may not adequately assess how decisions affect other divisions or the company as a whole; moreover, there is greater potential for duplication of duties, tasks, and initiatives if there is a lack of communication among teams or units.

Complicating the issue is the fact that the status of physical therapy practice, regardless of whether it is in a hospital setting or private practice, is often modified by macroeconomic or microeconomic crises. A recession or a change in the health care delivery paradigm, such as the change from fee-for-service to managed care reimbursement and the potential for "pay for performance" initiatives in the future, will affect the organizational structuring of the business. An organizational structure may also change as a result of internal crises, such as the sudden loss of a leader, a buy out from a larger stakeholder, or pressure to maintain a share of the market with stronger **competition**.

Nonetheless, the physical therapy practice that is efficient, effective, and adaptable in serving clients and able to effectively work within the constraints of organizational goals, competing demands, technological advances, and an ever-changing health care environment will be successful. The art and science of a stable organizational structure relies on the following:

- Efficiency: Reduce or eliminate wasted efforts or needless redundancies; divide work that is best managed through differentiation and coordinate work that needs integration; be responsive to the needs of clients and stakeholders in a timely fashion.
- Effectiveness: Ensure that all essential functions of each task are adequately addressed; distribute workload with consideration of optimal individual performance; optimize worker accountability through clear role delineation and expectations; create policies, procedures, and rules that work while minimizing conflict; use the most appropriate authority and power structure for your business (centralized or decentralized); clearly communicate goals.
- Adaptability: Balance rigidity in structure with productive creativity; foster collaboration while ensuring autonomy; measure effectiveness through outcome assessment and develop strategies based on valid information; use a well-founded strategy to continuously assess and revise goals.

EXERCISE 1-2

In a classroom setting, break into small groups (3-8 people). The following group/classroom discussion should be confidential. Confidentiality is recommended because the information disclosed has the potential of breaching the privacy of a patient care facility. Whenever possible, facility names should be kept anonymous. Discuss which of the characteristics of a classic bureaucracy apply to health care organizations in which participants work or have recently had clinical experience (you may even want to consider the physical therapy school in which you are currently enrolled). Explore which characteristics of the bureaucracy are deemed favorable, if any, and which are generally perceived as unfavorable in a physical therapy clinical environment. Justify the choices made. Discuss what physical therapy organizations, if any, might be appropriately labeled as bureaucracies. Share results, and discuss in the larger class setting.

Organizational Behavior

Organizational behavior refers to the way in which people interact, formally and informally, within business organizations. Understanding the behavior of individuals and groups within an organization assists in evaluating the impact of internal and external changes, predicting the behavior of workers faced with change, and adopting or adapting strategies in consideration of worker behaviors to better manage workers toward organizational goals. The sociologist Elton Mayo (1880-1949) recognized in 1927 that all business organizations, including health care and physical therapy practices, are social microsystems within which people interact and operate as groups to achieve common organizational goals. Mayo developed a human relations behavioralist management philosophy that stressed valuing human inputs as indispensable for organizational success.

Expounding on the scientific management theory of Fredrick Taylor and the human relations behavioralist management philosophy of Elton Mayo, Douglas McGregor (1906-1964) addressed managers' beliefs about the human nature of workers in his concepts of Theory X and Theory Y.

In Theory X, which is occasionally referred to as an *autocratic* style of management, managers perceive their employees as lazy and irresponsible people who, because of their dislike for work, must be controlled by rewards and punishment.

In Theory Y, which is occasionally referred to as a *participative* style of management, managers perceive their employees as responsible, self-directed, and creative people who enjoy their work (Box 1-3).

Another theory that warrants acknowledgment is Theory Z, often referred to as the *Japanese management* style. Developed by William Ouchi (born in 1943) and based on the work of Edward Deming (1900-1993), Theory Z purports that managers perceive workers as having discipline, a moral obligation to work hard, and a sense of collegiality. According to this system, which is based on trust, workers perform their jobs while managers support them and are concerned for their well-being (see Box 1-3). Although defining organizational behavior by theories is informative and can assist a manager in understanding organizations, a more pragmatic approach would be to thoroughly analyze the current or developing social microsystems within an organization. One approach takes into consideration the four Cs of organizational behavior: culture, climate, change, and communication. Becoming knowledgeable about the four Cs and developing short-term and long-term strategies based on this knowledge can lead to sustained success of the business.

Merriam-Webster's Collegiate Dictionary (ed 11) defines *culture* as "the set of shared attitudes, **values**, goals, and practices that characterizes an institution."[39] *Culture* refers to the enduring shared values and beliefs of the managers and workers that bond organization members together and contribute to the cohesive functioning of the company. Physical therapists typically seek employment with an organization that resonates well with their values and beliefs. In other words,

BOX **1-3** ■ **Comparison of Management Theories X, Y, and Z**

Management Theory X	Management Theory Y	Management Theory Z
• The most efficient organizations use a system of rewards and sanctions based on employee performance and a piece-rate pay system to optimize production and output. • Effective managers must scientifically analyze every aspect of every employee job, scientifically select their employees, closely supervise their employees to ensure that they employ scientific work methods, and constantly refine work processes scientifically.	• The most efficient organizations use a system of participative management wherein employees become personally involved in the organization and are involved in the decision-making process. • Effective managers must encourage creativity, ingenuity, and imagination of workers in shared decision making and an open management process.	• The most efficient organizations use a system of participative management wherein employees build co-operative and intimate working relationships with managers and co-workers, in which workers are well-trained generalists who are knowledgeable about the intricacies of the company's operations. • Effective managers must have a high degree of confidence in workers and promote high productivity standards, high employee morale, and satisfaction, thereby creating loyal and stable employees.

physical therapists seek a culture that is conducive to maximizing their potential to thrive in employment. Likewise, the initial perception of the employee about the organization and people working within it may determine how productive and satisfied that employee becomes and whether he or she remains with the organization. Some physical therapy clinics and American Physical Therapy Association chapters have developed mentorship programs or policies to assist with acclimation and transition into the organizational culture.

A first step in understanding a physical therapy practice culture would be to review the organization's mission, values statement, **vision statement**, goals/**objectives**, and standards of conduct or code of ethics. A review of these documents assists in the understanding of the enduring culture of the organization.

The second and more complicated step is to understand the interaction among individuals in the group with regard to roles and norms. An understanding of group dynamics is essential to an understanding of the culture. However, organizational culture should not be viewed as static because internal and external change can significantly influence the organization. Just as a significant life event can have a profound effect on the beliefs of an individual and ultimately affect his or her values, a significant change or event in the life of an organization can drastically change the organization's climate and ultimately the culture.

Climate refers to the current attitudes and perceptions of the managers and workers in relation to recent, perceived, inevitable, or potential internal and external changes. *Merriam-Webster's Collegiate Dictionary* defines *climate* as "the prevailing influence or environmental conditions characterizing a group or period."[39] Unlike culture, the organizational climate can change rather quickly. An internal change, such as losing or hiring a charismatic leader, or an external change, such as a significant revision in Medicare reimbursement, can affect the operations of the company and drastically change the organizational climate. Just as the study of the roles and norms of the group can provide insight into the organization's culture, a study of the cohesiveness of the group during times of change can contribute to the understanding of the organization's climate. Through relationships among managers and workers, who are organized into functional units or teams, members are expected to influence other members with regard to the accomplishment of shared goals. Group solidarity, cooperation, support, and ability to unite members toward shared goals are overt signs of cohesion and typically indicate a positive climate. Likewise, external factors that influence the stability of the organization and the degree of change required to maintain that relative stability have a major impact on the organizational climate. Being highly malleable, climate has an intimate relationship with change.

Most experienced clinicians can detail the accounts of a change in leadership or ownership that drastically altered their organization's climate or culture. The ability to initiate, accommodate, and optimize desired outcomes during change in an organization is essential for continued success of the business. Change, regardless of whether it is perceived as good or bad, is a challenge to all employees because it typically requires altering comfortable patterns of performance or habitual tendencies. Resistance to change is to be expected and can manifest itself in many ways, including but not limited to apathy, avoidance, passive-aggressive behavior, confrontations, discontent with policy and procedures, interpersonal conflicts, strain on collegiality, intradepartmental and interdepartmental conflicts, as well as covert and overt manipulation of the change process. Change is a phenomenon that unfolds over time at varying rates, with varying levels of control, and can be assessed in terms of quality and quantity. Uncontrolled organizational change involves a transformation in the organization that was initiated without the power or authority of those who manage the organization and as a result of external forces influencing operations or outcomes. Uncontrolled change is typically managed by reactionary measures and requires leadership and critical decision making for successful management. Controlled organizational change involves a transformation in the organization that is initiated by those who hold power or authority in the organization and may be the result of predicted, real, or perceived internal or external forces influencing operations. Controlled change can be preparatory, strategic, or reactionary. Controlled change is typically managed through individual and group influence or **strategic planning**. Prochaska and DiClemente identified six stages of how people change that are relevant to controlled organizational change.[42] The stages include precontemplation, contemplation, preparation, action, maintenance, and termination. The stages of change that occur in individuals can be applied to groups or organizations to assess the level of acceptance and action in adapting to internal and external influences on the business. A healthy physical therapy practice must always negotiate change for positive outcomes. Practices that are not proactive and reactive to the ever-changing health care market will be less likely to survive.

The key factor that maintains the functional structure of the organization is communication. Communication is the central organizing process of an organization that goes beyond sending and receiving messages through formal and informal lines of communication to making critical choices during interactions requiring interpersonal skills, such as being fully present in the moment, an active listener, and a reflective thinker. Formal lines of communication adhere to the organizational hierarchy of the business and require subordinates to approach the appropriate superior with comments, questions, or concerns. Likewise, a manager must communicate with the appropriate subordinate when delegating a specific task. In a more bureaucratic structure, the formal lines of communication are viewed as the most efficient avenue to perform work and accomplish goals. Formal lines of communication are established to reduce inaccuracies from second-hand information and result in problems being addressed by those who have the most authority and resources to resolve problems. Informal lines of communication are just as influential as formal lines of communication in affecting the climate of the organization. Opinion leaders, regardless of formal position, can influence the climate of an organization. Informal lines of communication are typically viewed as less efficient in terms of productivity because the information is second hand and does not address the problems to those who have the authority to make decisions, yet informal lines of communication can be more powerful than formal ones in affecting the climate of the organization. Nonetheless, when informal lines of communication are effectively used, efficiency can be improved through bypassing red tape and communicating with individuals who have the knowledge, expertise, or resources to solve a specific problem. Informal lines of communication are typically called grapevines for the way in which the communication weaves in and out of social networks of workers and managers. The grapevine can be influential in either open or closed organizational designs.

Although in-person communication is viewed as the best approach to minimizing miscommunication, the advent of other avenues of communication, such as telecommunication via cell phones, voice mail, conference calls, facsimile, email, and text messaging, are adding efficiency in disseminating information. Other modes of communication will continue to be optimized through technology, increasing the speed at which information is passed from one individual to another. Along with the rapid transfer of information come added complications, which we are just beginning to experience. New modes of communication can contribute to information overload and problems with information accuracy, truthfulness, and reliability. Too much information is difficult to process and filter for use, and false information can be quickly disseminated. No matter whether the misinformation was intentional or unintentional, it can be propagated quickly through formal and informal lines of communication and become the basis for faulty decision making. Managers should always validate the accuracy, truthfulness, credibility, trustworthiness, and reliability of the information used in decision making.

Understanding the four Cs of organizational behavior in the physical therapist's practice assists in directing workers toward organizational goals. The four Cs are related so that if a manager understands the *culture* and current *climate* of the organization, he or she can modify *communication* in order to effect a positive *change*. Likewise, when change is imposed on the organization, knowledge of the culture and tone of the climate can influence communication, assuming the manager works diligently to communicate in a manner that reduces conflict. Given that the pivotal factor in gaining positive outcomes is communication, a closer look at interpersonal communication and conflict negotiation, and **mediation**, is warranted.

EXERCISE 1-3

In a classroom setting, break into small groups (3-8 people). The following group/classroom discussion should be confidential. Confidentiality is recommended because the information disclosed has the potential of breaching the privacy of a patient care facility. Whenever possible, facility names should be kept anonymous. Discuss the characteristics of an organizational culture (e.g., shared attitudes, values, goals, practices) in which participants work or have recently had clinical experience. Independently rate the organizational climate on the following visual analog scale. Discuss, provide anecdotal evidence, and justify your ratings.

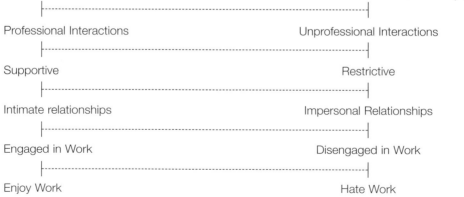

Professional Interactions	Unprofessional Interactions
Supportive	Restrictive
Intimate relationships	Impersonal Relationships
Engaged in Work	Disengaged in Work
Enjoy Work	Hate Work

EXERCISE 1-4

1. Review the foundational documents of your school or business organization (e.g., mission, values statement, vision statement, goals/objectives, standards of conduct or code of ethics). How would you describe the culture of this organization?
2. Assess the organizational climate of your classroom or work environment. From your evaluation of foundational documents, does the climate resonate with the stated mission and values? Is the climate conducive to achieving the vision? Develop a list of descriptors that characterize the current climate of your classroom or work environment.
3. Compare your findings with classmates or co-workers.

CONFLICT MANAGEMENT: COMMUNICATION AND NEGOTIATION

Interpersonal communication plays a pivotal role in business management and conflict management. Successful conflict management centers on the appropriate use of power and the application of negotiation tactics, which begins with interpersonal discourse. Through conversations, the physical therapist manager or staff physical therapist can influence decisions in a company by influencing the behaviors of others, as well as accomplish such tasks as gaining patient adherence to treatment protocols and gaining staff support of initiatives, while creating a rapport with colleagues or patients.

On the most basic level, in order to be competent at communication, the physical therapist manager or staff physical therapist must be attentive to and mindful of the other person during each interaction and provide appropriate expressiveness both verbally and nonverbally to develop understanding while creating or managing an effective rapport. The intended outcome of the interaction should remain the focus of the communication. One challenge is to keep one's mind from wandering from the current interaction by making a conscious effort to orient oneself to the conversation during discourse. Everyone is capable of processing multiple sensory inputs while entertaining various thoughts in a matter of seconds, and training is required to hone the skill of focusing on the interaction.

Another challenge is to closely monitor and appropriately interpret the other person's verbal and nonverbal cues. When the physical therapist is mindful of verbal communication, he or she takes into account the content, variations in language, tone, pitch, and pace of the other's verbalizations. Taking mental note of these elements can lead to important insights into the emotional undertones of the discourse. Physical therapists who are sensitive to nonverbal forms of communication take into account gestures, timing, use of touch, facial expressions, use of space, and artifacts such as dress and office arrangement when interpreting intent. It is important to listen attentively to and develop understanding from what the other person is saying before developing a response. Critically thinking about what has been said is also essential when considering the potential result of a response.

While engaged in communication, each participant should remain mindful of how less salient factors play a role in competent communication. Examples of these factors include issues of the past (e.g., experience, education, relationships), present (e.g., orientation, knowledge at hand, framing of the conversation, timing, an individual's power), and future (e.g., goals, agendas, strategic plans, positioning, expectations, predictions, forecasts). With all of these considerations being enacted in a matter of seconds, it is no wonder that much of what is communicated is misinterpreted and has the potential to cause conflict. Communication is a skill that every manager needs to continuously improve and maintain. Even those who are viewed as very competent communicators require practice to hone the skill; even when the skills are well established, occasional communication episodes can be viewed as incompetent. Because of the fluidness of discourse and ever-changing contexts, it is virtually impossible to always be competent in communication interactions, but the greater the knowledge of the variables affecting the situation, the better the potential outcome of the communication.

One important variable to consider when conflict is present during an interaction is the exchange of power. Power must be managed for a desirable outcome. Both the manager and employee have varying amounts of power to employ during the interaction. Power is the ability to influence another person's thoughts or actions in accordance with the possessor's wants or needs. At any given moment during an interaction, the manager or employee can construct and exert power that is either confirmed or contested by the other participant in the interaction. Power is, of course, constrained by the values and ethics of an organization, and even by the personal values, ethics, and morals of individuals within the organization. Despite their superior job titles or positions, managers do not necessarily have the power to control the interaction. As John French and Betram Raven claimed, individuals can possess reward power, coercive power, legitimate power, referent power, or expert power (or some combination thereof).[21] Each participant in an interaction can exert influence through the power of intrinsic and extrinsic rewards (e.g., creating a good reputation, receiving bonuses, improving productivity) or punishments (e.g., decreasing productivity, damaging the work climate, resisting the completion of tasks), as well as legitimate power (based on the cultural acceptance of traditional authority given by a particular role or position), referent power in the ability to create good rapport with others, and expert power derived from knowledge in a particular area. Power differentials cannot be ignored. Because of their formal positions, managers can exert greater control than their employees, but employee queries are seldom ignored because productivity depends on the employees. Likewise, the referent power of employees and the use of informal lines of communication can significantly influence the operation of a company. Controlling the interaction through the use of power has a significant influence on the outcomes of negotiation.

Negotiation is the foundation of conflict management. Negotiation is an exchange of information with an attempt to persuade or develop understanding among disputing parties to obtain a settlement. A mutually successful negotiation results in a settlement that is acceptable to all parties involved. However, many negotiations can result in different degrees of satisfaction among the parties involved, and typically the individual with less power at the time of the negotiation is less satisfied with the outcome. Critical thinking throughout the negotiation process is important. Negotiators should gather and analyze information (preferably before negotiation begins), critically analyze new information while problem solving during the interaction, and create a feasible resolution close to the preferred outcome. The problem-solving process in negotiation is not unlike the physical therapy evaluation in that the manager must gather subjective information and then examine objective findings. This evaluative process facilitates a thorough assessment of the situation and ultimately results in a plan for resolution. Nonetheless, intended goals may differ, as sometimes occurs between patients and therapists, and certain strategies must be employed to influence the negotiation. The first step is to develop bargaining objectives and establish a concrete range of acceptable options. The second step is to assume a mindset to optimize outcomes in good faith through negotiation with proper etiquette and a display of mutual respect. The third step is to select and appropriately employ conflict management strategies.

A common instrument used to assess conflict management strategies is the Thomas-Kilmann Conflict Mode Instrument.[47] Kenneth Thomas and Ralph Kilmann identified five different modes of addressing conflict: collaboration, **compromise**, **accommodation**, competition, and **avoiding**. Basing their theory on the Managerial Grid Model developed by Robert Blake and Jane Mouton,[11] Thomas and Kilmann focused on the degree of concern for people versus the concern for task completion to determine the mode of conflict resolution utilized. Collaboration, sometimes considered a negotiation technique used to arrive at a *win-win situation*, occurs when the parties involved in the conflict exchange information openly, seek solutions that are acceptable to everyone involved, and work together without becoming entrenched in an opinion. Arriving at a solution through collaboration typically takes time and energy, but the participants have a high regard for one another and are assertive in satisfying their own concerns for task completion. Compromise, sometimes referred to as "reaching a middle ground," requires that the participants in the conflict define the concessions that each party is willing to make to resolve the conflict. The defining difference between collaboration and compromise is that the participants involved in compromise have taken a particular stance on the resolution of the conflict. A compromise is more likely to occur when the goals of the participants are mutually exclusive, participant power has been equalized, and participants are committed to resolving the issue without a stalemate. Accommodation is a resolution of conflict in which the opposing participant's request is granted. When a manager reaches a resolution through accommodation, he or she cooperates while suppressing an attempt to satisfy his or her own concerns. A mode of conflict resolution that is considered opposite to accommodation is competition. Competition, also known as a *win-lose situation*, requires all parties involved to be assertive in the use of their power with less or no regard for satisfying the others' concerns. The individual with the most power in the conflict situation will move forward with his or her resolution of the conflict. This strategy is typically employed when a decision must be made quickly, there is a perceived need to protect one's self-interest, or the resolution of the conflict is vital to the company. The final mode of conflict management addressed by Thomas and Kilmann is avoiding. Avoiding, sometimes viewed as an opposite to collaboration, is a strategy of withdrawing from the conflict. Avoidance is typically used when there is a fear of being in a position of lower power, when the issue is not important to the participant, or when the issue can be resolved by others. Avoidance may also be used as a strategy to allow time for the intensity of the conflict to diminish or for additional information to be gathered, or when the cost of engaging in the conflict outweighs the benefit of resolving the conflict. The appropriate use of any and all strategies depends on reflective analysis and response to a particular situation. Physical therapy managers should not develop rules for when to use a strategy but should instead become proficient enough to use each strategy appropriately for the desired outcome. They should always weigh the consequences of initiating a specific strategy before implementation.

Physical therapy managers who are interested in a conflict management tool that takes into account shifts in stress levels and cultural sensitivity should refer to the Kraybill Conflict Style Inventory.[35] Ron Kraybill identified five styles of responding to conflict (i.e., directing, harmonizing, avoiding, cooperating, and compromising), a schema that accounts for varying responses in "calm" and "storm" conditions and differentiates responses on the basis of whether the user comes from a collectivist- as opposed to an individualist-oriented culture.

Negotiation is a term that can be used in interpersonal relationships, such as negotiating the perception of our identity, in addition to legal contexts, wherein two individuals negotiate a contract. In a broader sense, negotiation is considered a subcategory of alternative dispute resolution (ADR). When a third party becomes involved in the resolution of a conflict, the terms *mediation* or **arbitration** are used. Mediation is when a third party helps to negotiate a resolution by bringing the parties in dispute closer to a mutual and fair resolution. In arbitration the third party is given the power to adjudicate or impose a solution on the parties in dispute. For further information on mediation, refer to "Model of Standards of Conduct for Mediators," created collaboratively by the American Bar Association, the American Arbitration Association, and the Association for Conflict Resolution (2005).[4]

Negotiations inherently involve conflict between individuals or among members of groups. Physical therapy managers frequently work through the process of negotiation. The manager will also have opportunities to mediate or arbitrate conflict between employees, often without prior training. In professional settings, such as physical therapy practices, disagreement cannot be permitted to fester into disenchantment, which results in diminished quality of patient care services. Substantive disagreements, as well as introduction of material changes in policies or procedures, must be aired openly among staff members. Formalized negotiation processes optimize the flow and outcomes of such events.

EXERCISE 1-5

Divide into labor and management teams; use the information on conflict management to prepare for negotiating the issues in the case scenarios below; then bargain over this issue to conclusion (time commitment 1-6 hours). The course instructor should act as facilitator and create confidential information for each team to use in the exercise.

CASE 1

ABC Health System is a leading community hospital in a midsize Northeast city. ABC has three competitors, all of which recently implemented 7-day comprehensive (full-service) rehabilitation coverage for their inpatients and outpatients. ABC is unionized throughout the system, and the rank-and-file have strong resistance to moving from 5- to 7-day full coverage. Good luck!

CASE 2

IBCore Medical System operates in the western half of a large rust-belt state, controlling some 150 clinical sites and employing more than 450 physical therapists, physical therapist assistants, and support and administrative staff. IBCore wants to dominate physical therapy service delivery throughout the region of five nearby states. To do so in the eyes of the Chairman requires, among other things, a federal contract to provide physical therapy services in federal facilities within these five states. To be competitive for such a contract with the current conservative executive governmental team, the following are deemed essential for IBCore to have in place: (1) a drug awareness program for compliance with the federal Drug-Free Workplace Act and (2) a comprehensive employee drug-testing program. The employees of IBCore are unionized and are adamantly opposed to workplace drug testing. (Before starting, read the drug-testing vignette below.) Good luck!

Drug-Free Workplace Act of 1988

The Drug-Free Workplace Act of 1988[19] requires that companies and individuals who enter into contracts with the federal government, valued at $25,000 or more, certify that their facilities are drug-free workplaces. Federal contractors are required, at least, to do the following:

- Have in place an effective workplace drug education program
- Post and give to each employee a copy of the prohibition against the "unlawful manufacture, distribution, [use], or [possession] of controlled substances ... in the workplace,"[18] specifying potential disciplinary actions for violation of the prohibition
- Notify the federal contracting agency, within 10 days, of any drug-related criminal convictions of its employees

The Drug-Free Workplace Act of 1988 does not specifically mandate that employers carry out workplace drug testing; however, neither are they prohibited by the statute from doing so.

Workplace drug testing is of relatively recent vintage. It first began in the military during the 1970s. By 1983, 3% of companies in the United States carried out workplace drug testing. Currently, about one third of Fortune 500 corporations test their employees for illicit drug use.[16] Employee drug testing includes the following tests[1]:

- Pre-employment drug screening, the most commonly used employee drug test type: Pre-employment drug testing is recognized as a common law management right to promote an employer's legitimate business interests.
- Reasonable-suspicion drug testing, performed when a supervisor of an employee reasonably believes that the employee may be under the influence of mind-altering drugs: Legal bases for reasonable-suspicion drug testing include the fact that employers are vicariously liable for the conduct of employees acting within the scope of employment and the statutory requirement under the Occupational Safety and Health Act of 1970 for employers to maintain a workplace free of serious safety hazards.
- Periodic drug testing of employees, such as during a periodic physical examination or as part of a promotion to a position that requires the employee to handle classified documents or carry a firearm
- Post-accident drug testing, after serious accidents, with or without suspicion of employee misconduct
- Random drug testing, the least often used and most effective and controversial form of employee drug testing
- Exculpatory drug testing,[44] designed to exculpate an employee who erroneously tests positive for illicit drug use by comparing the blood types of the suspect and blood group substances found in the positive urine sample. Approximately 80% of the population are "secretors" of such substances, for whom exculpatory testing, based on ABO blood groups, is feasible.

Case law to date addressing the constitutionality and propriety of employee drug testing has generally upheld the practice, with one proviso. Except for military service members and prisoners, direct observation of a subject rendering a urine sample is universally considered to be repugnant and an unconscionably impermissible violation of personal human dignity and privacy. In business settings, therefore, only indirect observation of subjects rendering urine samples is permitted, such as the posting of a guard outside of a lavatory so that extraneous paraphernalia is not carried in by testees.

Effective January 1, 1996, all transit employers regulated by the U.S. Department of Transportation (DOT) were required to have, in addition to drug awareness programs, alcohol abuse prevention programs that comply with DOT's specific regulations. These federal regulations preempt any conflicting state laws concerning alcohol misuse. Safety-sensitive employees, including truck and bus drivers, are prohibited from imbibing alcohol 4 hours before driving and are subject to testing to confirm that they are free of alcohol and other drugs while on the job.[2]

MANAGEMENT AND LEADERSHIP

As an old adage states, "Anyone can manage, but not everyone can lead." Management is an administrative, bureaucratic function, in which an appointed superior orders subordinates to carry out duties associated with their employment. A manager is someone situated in a position of relative authority on an organizational chart who conducts the activities of a business, department, or unit. Like a manager, a director must carry out the organizing, motivating, and supervising of employees, but the director is entrusted with the additional responsibility of directing the future course of the business, department, or unit. Some organizations use the titles of manager and director synonymously. Managers can learn their roles and functions through informal training on the job or through formal education. Likewise, directors can learn to articulate a vision and develop strategies to move in a particular direction. Nonetheless, without leadership to maintain operations, assist employees in coping with change, and inspire employees to meet a shared goal, the organization is at risk of inefficiency and low productivity.

A leader is one who compels subordinates and others to action through inspiration and motivation. A leader is a catalyst to desired action who often, but not always, occupies a position of authority on an organizational chart. According to Kraemer, characteristics of a manager include short-range involvement, good problem-solving skills and deductive reasoning, the ability to work well within the system, a convergent thinking style, and relative passivity.[34] A leader possesses some of these characteristics but also some additional ones, such as long-range inspiration, innovation, inductive reasoning skills, empowerment of others, a divergent thinking style, and a predisposition to act proactively. A leader is visionary, inspirational, and practical, according to Isaacson and Ford.[32] He or she must not only develop a well-crafted vision for the organization but also effectively communicate that vision and organizational goals and objectives to the members, inspiring them to embrace these priorities as their own. Goffee and Jones believe that a leader must also show his or her human side by selectively revealing weaknesses to others and freely revealing differences of opinion with others in the organization.[24] The concept of power, as discussed earlier, intricately relates to management authority and leadership. Power is a relational phenomenon and the essence of leadership. A leader has the ability to wield power in various situations. But are these characteristics a part of nature (i.e., leadership skill that is a genetic predisposition) or nurture (i.e., skills that potential leaders can learn)?

The industrial revolution of the early 1900s spawned various theories of leadership. Beginning with "great person" and trait theories and evolving to more contemporary theories of transformational, visionary, and service leadership, the literature reflects the continued attempt to operationally define effective leadership. Researchers continue to search for a unifying theory of leadership for application in various contexts. As empiricism and the scientific method became the basis of gaining knowledge, behavioral theories of leadership became the predominant approach to studying leadership in the early 1900s to mid 1960s. During this era, leadership research focused on characteristics and traits that are inherent in leaders.

One of the most well-known behavioral models, the Managerial Grid Model, discussed earlier in this chapter, informed the TKI and Kraybill conflict inventories. This model, by Blake and Mouton, implemented a grid in which concern for people was indicated on the vertical axis and concern for task was indicated on the

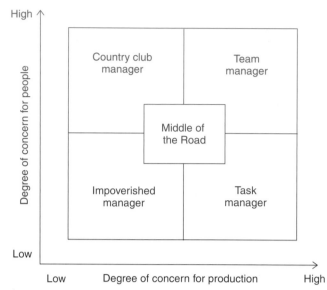

FIGURE 1-1 | Managerial grid model. (Managerial Grid adapted courtesy Grid International, Austin, Texas.)

horizontal axis.[11] The bottom left corner of the grid was termed "impoverished management," denoting a leader who would exert minimal effort to accomplish work and demonstrate little concern for people or the task. A higher concern for task and lower concern for people was termed an "authority-compliance" or task manager management style. A high concern for people and low concern for task was called "country club management"; this style was viewed as relatively friendly but inefficient in terms of task completion. A high concern for people and task was viewed as optimal and termed "team management." Blake and Mouton also considered a "middle of the road" management style, placed in the middle of the grid, which was less efficient than team management but still suited to accomplishing the task while demonstrating a concern for people (Figure 1-1).

Continuing the search for characteristics or traits of leadership, the Ohio State Leadership Studies, conducted during the 1940s, identified the following common traits*:

• Physical vitality and stamina
• Intelligence and action-oriented judgment
• Eagerness to accept responsibility
• Task competence
• Understanding of followers and their needs
• Skill in dealing with people

---

*From Gardner J: *On leadership*, New York, 1989, Free Press.

- Need for achievement
- Courage and resolve
- Trustworthiness
- Decisiveness
- Self-confidence
- Assertiveness
- Adaptability/flexibility

Also classified as behavioral approaches to leadership are the participative leadership styles of Lewin and Likert. Lewin's research in 1939 using decision experiments identified three styles of leadership: autocratic, democratic, and laissez-faire.[36] The autocratic style of leader makes decisions without consulting members, whereas the democratic style of leader involves members in decision making. The laissez-faire leader allows members to make decisions for themselves without a centralized control of the initiatives. In 1967, Rensis Likert considered the degree to which members are involved in decision making, identifying four distinct styles of leadership: exploitive authoritative, benevolent authoritative, consultative, and participative.[37] An exploitive authoritative leadership style uses coercive reinforcement to gain compliance, whereas the benevolent authoritative style focuses on rewarding members for compliance. In consultative leadership, the leader seeks input from the members but still controls decisions. The participative leadership style uses a low power differential to maximize member input into decisions.

Realizing that most behavioral theories did not take into account the contextual situation, which is considered an essential variable in leadership, researchers turned to contingency theories in the 1960s to 1980s. Fiedler's **contingency theory** of leadership, the first contribution to this approach, systematically accounted for situational factors.[20] The contingency theory holds that a leader's ability to exert influence over others, which is variable across organizations and is situation dependent, determines group effectiveness. Through aligning leadership style with the favorableness of the situation, Fiedler proposes an analysis of the leader-member relationship, the structure and orientation to the task at hand, and the leader's power in the situation as a requisite in determining or predicting group effectiveness.

In the 1970s, a class of contingency theories called *situational leadership* developed. Hersey and Blanchard provide a good example of how such contingency models work.[28] Their leadership model is one of the most widely known subordinate-centered leadership approaches to date. Applying the model in a physical therapy context, consider how a physical therapist's leadership style may change as an employee's knowledge, skills, and level of expectations increase. Basing their conclusions on the maturity of the individuals being led and the stability of an organization, Hersey and Blanchard delineate four possible approaches to leadership: **directive** leadership, which is low in support but high in direction to subordinates; **coaching**, high both in support and direction; **delegating**, low in both support and direction; and **supporting**, which is high in support but low in direction. In sum, directive and coaching forms of leadership are relatively hands-on. A student physical therapist in the clinic begins in a highly directive relationship with his or her clinical instructor, whereas a new graduate physical therapist in his or her first month at the job may receive coaching from another physical therapist mentor until comfortable with the procedures of the clinic. Delegating and supporting approaches to leadership are relatively hands-off. Once the clinical instructor is assured of the student's competence (e.g., after the student has passed an examination), the instructor will take a supportive role during an evaluation. Similarly, once the new graduate has worked in the setting for more than a month or so, the physical therapist manager can delegate a full patient load to the new therapist. Acknowledging that this model is oversimplified, we can easily give examples of leaders becoming proficient at or using a preferred style predominantly with good results. Consider the difference in leadership styles exemplified by two United States presidents: Jimmy Carter and Ronald Reagan. The former was considered a highly hands-on micromanager and the latter was often labeled the "great delegator." Arguably, both leaders were equally effective. Physical therapist managers can easily apply this situational leadership model to situations in practice.

Influenced by the Ohio State Leadership Studies and expectancy theories of motivation, Robert House proffered a model called the *path-goal theory of leadership,* under which leader behavior is defined according to how the leader positively affects subordinates' performance and their effect on organizational goals and objectives.[30] House labeled leadership styles as directive, supportive, participative, and achievement-oriented. The contingency variables in the path-goal theory are environment and member characteristics that influence leader behaviors and ultimately outcomes. Just before House developed his path-goal theory, Vroom, Yetton, and Jago defined leadership by selecting the best alternative and subordinate participation or acceptance of the desired action.[49] Their leader-participation model defined decision procedures, including autocratic (with and without information sharing), consultative (in person and impersonal in nature), and group decision-making (consensus agreement). Tannenbaum and Schmidt's Continuum of Leadership Behavior was developed through research on the need to evaluate situational factors before using a leadership style.[46] Their continuum ranges from boss-centered leadership to subordinate-centered leadership, and situational factors determine which approach is appropriate. Throughout the continuum, managers consider options of appropriate member involvement in decision making on the basis of the situation at hand.

In an era of constant change in health care delivery systems and processes, contingency approaches to leadership and management are probably most widely understood and used by physical therapy managers. Health care managers can easily gravitate toward approaches that are situational in nature, proactive, and highly fluid. Leadership books, primarily those based on contingency approaches for the lay public, are quite popular. Although relevant insight can be gleaned from such books, most physical therapy managers quickly realize that one approach is not necessarily preferable, because there simply is no single "best" way to lead or manage people.

Behavioral and contingency theories contain a good deal of valuable information; however, the theories tend to oversimplify. Management of today's physical therapy practices warrants a consideration of contemporary leadership theories. Building on the knowledge of behavioral, participative, situational, and other contingency theories of leadership, current scholars are exploring transactional and transformational leadership theories. Based on behavioralism, including classical and operant conditioning, transactional theories work on the contingency of motivation produced by punishment or rewards. Transactional leaders attempt to create clear formal structures and well-defined roles for the leader and members. Contractual agreements between managers and members provide authority to leaders for a "management by exception" orientation. Management by exception empowers managers to actively search for deviations from the set rules or passively monitor whether standards are being met and take corrective action when needed. The most prevalent transactional theory of leadership, with a greater concentration on interpersonal influences and leader-member relationship, is the Leader-Member Exchange Model.[25,26] The Leadership-Member Exchange Model (LMX; also known as the *Vertical Dyad Linkage Theory*) emphasizes the exchange of personal and positional resources, or tacit agreements, in order to maintain a leadership role and optimize the performance of members. Based on a continuum from high LMX (i.e., mutual trust and low power differential) to low LMX (i.e., formal authority and high power differential), leader-member relationships are analyzed. The LMX process begins when a member joins the organization and takes a defined role according to his or her position and the leader's assessment of the member's abilities. The second step of the process is an informal negotiation of becoming part of the in-group (with the leader) or the out-group. The in-group member provides dedication and loyalty to the leader in exchange for benefits, such as increased power or extrinsic rewards (e.g., merit raise, interesting duties, greater autonomy). Conversely, an out-group member performs the duties that he or she was hired to perform but is given low levels of autonomy or influence in the job. The final step, termed *routinization*, is a relatively stable pattern of social exchange between the leader and member.

Whereas a transactional leader manages by use of goal setting, rules, standards, clarifying roles, task delineation, and established routines of behavior, a transformational leader seeks to inspire members to transcend their own self-interests for the good of the organization. Inspiring members to a sense of mission and clear vision for the organization, the transformational leader gives individualized attention to members while creating respect, trust, and high expectations for performance. Bass's Transformational Leadership Theory emphasizes the need for leaders to create followers through charisma.[7] Followers are transformed from members through increased awareness of the importance of the tasks they perform, a focus on the organizational goals rather than on self-interests, and activation of higher-level needs, such as "esteem needs" or "self-actualization needs" on Abraham Maslow's Hierarchy of Needs or "motivational factors" in reference to Frederick Herzberg's Motivation Hygiene Theory.[29,38] Bass postulated that charisma is rooted in the moral character of the leader and the ethical value of the initiatives. He views transformational leadership as grounded in idealized influence, inspirational motivation, intellectual stimulation, and individualized consideration.[8] Burn's Transformational Leadership Model[15] focused on leaders and members inspiring one another to achieve higher levels of motivation and morality. Similarly, in his book *Good to Great* Jim Collins called transformational leadership "level 5 leadership."[17] He described transformational leaders as being in step with what the organization does best (i.e., hedgehog concept) and more focused on the organization's vision, the company, and the work than on their own self-interests.

James Kouzes and Barry Posner[33] made a significant contribution to transformational leadership theories by surveying more than 75,000 people about characteristics that would inspire them to follow a particular leader. In order of importance, people preferred to follow leaders who are honest, forward-thinking, competent, inspiring, intelligent, fair-minded, broad-minded, supportive, straightforward, dependable, cooperative, determined, imaginative, ambitious, courageous, caring, mature, loyal, self-controlled, and independent. By modeling these characteristics and enabling members to act, leaders become successful. In addition, Kouzes and Posner emphasized inspiring a shared vision, approaching challenges, and being passionate about one's work.

Through the survey research of David Rooke and William Torbert, seven developmental action logics were identified, providing a new emphasis in transformational leadership. Rooke and Torbert argued that it is how leaders "interpret their surroundings and react when their power or safety is challenged" that distinguishes leaders (e.g., a leader's "action logic").[43] Below-average performance of individuals and corporations was associated with leaders classified as opportunists, diplomats, and experts. An average performance was found in corporations with leaders classified as achievers, and high performance was associated with leaders demonstrating action logics of individualists, strategists, and alchemists. The developmental stages begin with the opportunist, who focuses on personal accomplishments and exploits others to further his or her own achievement. The diplomat is a person who seeks to please others, is self-conscious to the point of stifling his or her ability to control external events or members, and tends to avoid conflict while trying to maintain the status quo. The expert seeks knowledge to gain control over the environment and manage members of the organization. Experts tend to provide rational and logical arguments by presenting the facts with supporting data in attempts to gain member support. Achievers tend to focus on outcomes and create a positive work environment. They are team players who conform to rules but tend to have difficulty in thinking outside the box. An individualist tends to view the organization from a constructivist perspective, being aware that rules can be a hindrance to the accomplishment of intended outcomes, but nonetheless finds creative ways to accomplish outcomes. The strategist tends to focus on the organizational and situational constraints and perception to institute change through an iterative developmental process. Strategists are good at creating a shared vision and generating organizational transformations. At the highest level of development in transformations of leadership is the alchemist. According to Rooke and Torbert, the alchemist has the rare "ability to renew or even reinvent themselves and their organizations in historically significant ways."[43] The alchemist has the ability to multitask at various levels while addressing immediate priorities and without losing sight of intended outcomes.

Contemporary leadership theorists acknowledge the need for development of community in organizations. The success of the community depends on members and leaders. The theory founded on the interdependence of member and leader is servant leadership. The concept of servant leadership was developed in 1970 by Robert Greenleaf. However, the origin of servant leadership is said to have historical roots in the teaching of Jesus of Nazareth (8-2 BC/BCE–29-36 AD/CE) or even ancient Chinese scriptures such as the Tao Te Ching (estimated at 600 BCE). The focus of servant leadership is to maintain the organization's integrity while serving others. The principle followed by these leaders is to serve others first and then to provide further service through leadership. A high priority of servant leaders is the success of those whom he or she serves. The commonality among contemporary leadership models is an adherence to the core values and the ideological purpose of the organization. Regardless of the adopted leadership style of the manager, the alignment of the organization's values, mission, vision, goals and objectives in relation to the perpetual changes of the external environment of the business of health care must be appropriately managed.

To be a successful leader, the manager must have a comprehensive understanding of the organization, its culture, its climate, its people, and the environment in which productivity is achieved. Along with this understanding, a leader needs to engage in daily critical and reflective thinking, decisive decision making with consideration of future implications, and a vision of where the company should be moving in light of economic, political, technological, and health care trends. A new manager can learn about the organization through an analysis of its history, present environment, and future vision (Box 1-4).

The values of an organization are reflected in the **mission statement**. A mission statement defines why the organization exists. The mission statement provides a written identity to the organization by reflecting its core values, creating an image, emphasizing the quality of its employees, highlighting services offered and differentiating these services from those of other competing providers, and defining the population served. The mission statement typically includes general demographic information about the organization and the clients served (e.g., name, address, areas of expertise, services provided, target market, noted stakeholders) while creating a cohesive statement through integrating elements of the organization's core values, culture, and philosophies. A sample mission statement from Brooke Army Medical Center, San Antonio, Texas, appears below.[13]

> "To improve the health of our community while ensuring deployment readiness of Brooke Army Medical Center personnel. We do it by operating a customer-focused, quality-integrated health care system and by conducting graduate medical education and clinical investigation."

BOX **1-4** ▪ **Understanding Your Organization**

- As a start to learning about an organization, consider the core values of the physical therapy practice and what is considered its ideological core. Values represent strongly held beliefs, whereas an ideology sets the bar through a set of shared ideals and aspirations that members strive to achieve in their daily work. Search out the written and unwritten shared values of the practice. If a document of shared values does not exist, consider developing a list of shared values of the practice and writing a value statement, sometimes referred to as a *philosophical statement,* for the organization. Some suggestions and insights for managers to consider are listed below:
  - Every member of the physical therapy practice wants to work for a reputable and successful company; managers must ensure a solid reputation for the practice through professionalism and ethical behaviors in the service of others and build success through dedication to excellence and continuous quality improvement.
  - Values are instilled in employees from the time of hiring; managers must be role models, mentors, and educators to assist in establishing appropriate behaviors and organizational values in new employees.
  - Values are shared; managers must reward outward embodiment of shared values and discourage disruptive behaviors.
  - Values become ingrained in the employee but can be dramatically changed by significant events; in times of crisis, managers must maintain integrity through open and honest communication, accurately and honestly representing the situation at hand and following through on promises or obligations made to employees.
  - Each individual in the practice has an impact on the values of the practice; managers must recognize and respect the personal goals and varying needs of individual employees.
  - Employees bring personal core values to the practice that may or may not resonate with organizational core values; managers must thoroughly consider new hires and select the right people for the practice. On the other hand, managers must terminate employment of those members who are irreparably disruptive or in some way detrimental to maintaining the values of the business.

A driving force behind a mission statement is the vision statement. A vision statement is a projection of where the organization wants to be in regard to future development. The vision statement of a physical therapy practice provides a concise, vivid image of the organization's future identity and position in the health care market. Tying the vision statement to attainable goals leads to action plans focused on realizing the vision and inspiring workers.

The ability of the leader to make the vision realistic, attainable, adaptable, and ultimately perpetual depends on a feasible action plan with realizable goals and adequate resources to succeed. An action plan in business is typically called a

---

BOX **1-5** ▪ **Steps in Strategic Planning**

1. Glean a pragmatic understanding of the mission and vision.
2. Assess the environment.
3. Develop broad goals based on the mission, vision, and environmental assessment.
4. Develop objectives to achieve goals.
5. Weigh the costs and benefits of alternative strategies to meet objectives and select the most beneficial and feasible strategy.
6. Implement the chosen strategy in an appropriate and timely manner.
7. Use formative and summative evaluation and feedback to optimize goal attainment.

---

strategic plan. Although a strategic plan may have set time frames, strategic planning must be a continuous process to address the dynamics of the health care environment. Strategic planning is the process of defining the direction of an organization through delineating guidelines and designating a process to accomplish the vision (Box 1-5).

The first step is to review the mission and vision of the physical therapy practice. The mission statement should be relatively stable, enduring, and referred to often; however, it is a good practice to consider revision of a physical therapy practice mission statement every 5 to 7 years to reflect changes in the business and health care environments. The vision statement should be developed with the mission in mind and remain relevant for a period of 3 to 5 years or longer. The vision statement should be a common topic of discussion among employees and harmonious with the mission, goals, and strategies of the business.

The second step is to conduct a thorough assessment of environmental opportunities and constraints. A common approach to an environmental assessment is to consider the internal strengths and weaknesses of the business and external opportunities and threats (or barriers) affecting the business. This approach is called a SWOT (or SWOB) analysis (an acronym for strengths, weaknesses, opportunities, and threats [or barriers]). A SWOT analysis assists in assessing the internal and external environmental factors that have an impact on the physical therapy practice. Some common internal factors that may be identified as strengths or weaknesses include financial stability, personnel, facilities, material resources, and so on. Common external factors include competitors, changes in the economy, governmental health care regulation changes, third-party payer reimbursement changes, and other social or client influences. Two other approaches are occasionally used in businesses to perform an environmental audit: the five forces analysis and the PEST analysis.

Michael Porter developed the concepts underlying the five forces analysis and their impact on the **microenvironment** of businesses.[41] Microenvironmental influences are those factors that are specific to a practice's area of activity and directly affect the ability of the business to provide services and make a profit.

In application to a physical therapy practice, the five forces include identifying the following:

- The threat of entry; threats of beginning a physical therapy practice
- The power of buyers; power of clients making a choice of practitioners
- The power of suppliers; the power of other health care practices having an immovable market share of your potential clientele
- The threat of substitutes; the threat of other health care practices supplying similar services
- Degree of rivalry; the combined threat of other health care providers, similar service providers, and clients' choice on the attempts of the practice to gain a market share

Macroenvironmental influences are more general, external forces that affect the health care sector of business rather than an area of activity specific to the practice. PEST is an acronym for political forces, economic forces, sociocultural forces, and technological forces, all of which influence the organization's environment. These factors are considered to be less subject to control by the practice but are as influential as internal influences in the direction of a practice.

After assessment of the internal, microenvironmental, and macroenvironmental factors, the next step of the strategic plan is to develop well-defined goals and objectives. Because distinguishing between a goal and an objective is sometimes confusing, physical therapists can use an analogy related to writing short-term and long-term goals for patients. Short-term goals are comparable to objectives in the context of strategic planning. An objective is something tangible toward which the efforts of the business are directed. When objectives are accomplished, the result is closer proximity to the goal. An acronym commonly used in strategic planning and program evaluation is SMART objectives. In regard to patient care, physical therapists understand the importance of making SMART objectives because patient outcomes need to be specific, measurable, achievable, relevant, and time framed. In fact, some third-party payers will refuse payment if objectives (i.e., physical therapy goals) are not being met and written in a similar format to SMART objectives. In strategic planning, a goal is more visionary and focused on one area of desired accomplishment over a specific time frame. A goal should be achievable and realistic and clearly describe the vision of what the organization would like to accomplish. From a physical therapist's perspective, a strategic planning goal can be conceptualized as analogous to a physical therapy long-term goal for patient care.

The next step is to choose among available strategies to optimize achievement of objectives and goals. The choice of strategy must take into consideration all prior steps of strategic planning, with additional emphasis on the following:

- Availability and allocation of resources (e.g., financial, personnel, material)
- Selection of the right person or people to assign responsibility and accountability to complete the objective(s)
- Development of a verbal and written communication or reporting procedure
- Assessment of the influence of time available for accomplishment of objectives and development of a timeline to accomplish tasks

- A written plan detailing all components of the strategy (e.g., intent, resources, roles, responsibilities, desired outcomes, timeline, evaluation)
- Continuous management of the strategy process through ongoing examination and evaluation
- Attentiveness to the strategy from implementation to completion

Implementation of the selected strategy coincides with the initiation of examination and evaluation. The components of examination and evaluation are similar to the constructs in the *Guide to Physical Therapy Practice* patient/client management model.[3] Examination requires a gathering of information. An examination can contain brief, readily available data for quick feedback (also known as a **formative evaluation**) or detailed information gathered at designated points on a timeline. The detailed examination can include, but is not limited to, a history of the strategic plan, a review of the intent of the objectives and goals, the stage of plan implementation, accomplishment of objectives to date, accomplishments of members to date, barriers or hindrances to initiatives, adherence to timelines, utilization of resources, and so on. This thorough examination is typically used for a **summative evaluation**, which is focused on outcomes at a critical point in the strategic plan. Summative evaluation is intended to identify possible problems, assess performance of members, seek resolution to problems found, and appropriately adjust the strategic planning process to meet current needs and future expectations. A summative evaluation is often written and distributed to stakeholders, whereas a formative evaluation is intended to give timely feedback to guide, modify, or redirect the strategic plan toward the intended goal in light of developments.

A successful strategic plan depends primarily on the people and the planning. The members need to develop a vested interest in the success of the strategic plan, clearly understand their roles, and be held accountable for the responsibilities that they are assigned or have accepted (a transactional leader would say, "preferably through a written agreement or contract"). All stakeholders should be involved in the process to develop a strong communication network and to secure stakeholder buy-in. Inattentiveness of managers or members will derail the strategic plan as easily as overt or covert resistance. Inattentiveness can be due to apathy, indifference, poor organizational climate, multitasking, and duty overload, among other hindering factors. The strategic plan should align the values, vision, and mission of the company or department with its goals, objectives, and outcome measures (e.g., score cards, benchmarks, checklist of accomplishments). A well-structured plan should maintain a focus on goals while minimizing untimely shifting between competing goals. The plan should appropriately assess the competence of financial, material, and personnel resources; include strategies to optimize understanding and communication; and provide salient incentives for plan completion that match the participant efforts. Finally, the plan should be responsive to current needs and flexible enough to meet change with strategies that optimize goal completion; it should also be oriented to the future success of the business.

SUMMARY

The business organization is becoming increasingly complex. This statement especially applies to health care organizations, in which the only certainty is constant change. Clinical managers must be cognizant of organizational theories regarding open and closed organizations and assess which type they are managing. Organizational behavior, the processes under which co-workers interact, is critically important as well. Managers should pay special attention to organizational culture and climate and foster it through ceremonies, social functions, and other tangible and intangible means of promoting a collective identity within the work force. Managers must be leaders who are instrumental in change and operate proactively in support of organizational goals and objectives. Managers must demonstrate the careful use of power, or the ability to cause others to act, every day. The managerial skill of interpersonal negotiations is one of the most important, and managers should have a framework from which to successfully negotiate with others. Managers are role models for their workers and either inspire or alienate them. Managers, as leaders, must motivate employees to maintain a focused effort toward goal achievement. The accomplishment of goals depends on a sound strategic plan. Strategic planning incorporates the values, vision, and mission of the business while optimizing the vested interest of members in the completion of well-defined objectives and goals. The outcomes of an effective leader and well-founded strategic plan can ensure the future success of a physical therapy practice.

REFERENCES AND READINGS

1. Aalberts RJ, Rubin HW: A risk management analysis of employee drug abuse and testing, *Chartered Property and Casualty Underwriters Journal* 41(2): 105-111, 1988.
2. Allen TY: DOT Drug-Testing Rules Require Detailed Plans, *HR News*, March 1996, pp. 3, 9.
3. American Physical Therapy Association: Guide to physical therapy practice (ed 2), *Physical Therapy* 81(1): s31-s42, 2001.
4. American Bar Association, American Arbitration Association, and Association for Conflict Resolution: Model Standards of Conduct for Mediators. http://www.abanet.org/dispute/news/ModelStandardsofConductforMediatorsfinal05.pdf. (Retrieved August 10, 2006.)
5. Ainsworth-Vaughn N: *Claiming power in doctor-patient talk*, New York, 1998, Oxford University Press.
6. Bass BM: *Leadership and performance beyond expectations*, New York, 1985, Free Press.
7. Bass BM: From transactional to transformational leadership: learning to share the vision, *Organizational Dynamics* 19-31, Winter 1990.
8. Bass BM, Steidlmeier P: Ethics, character and authentic transformational leadership. http://cls.binghamton.edu/BassSteid.html. (Retrieved February 8, 2007.)
9. Bedeian A, Zammuto R: *Organizations theory and design*, Chicago, 1991, Dryden Press.
10. Blake R, Mouton J: *Group dynamics: Key to decision making*, Houston, 1961, Gulf Publishing Co.

11. Blake R, Mouton J: *The managerial grid*, Houston, 1964, Gulf Publishing Co.
12. Brady L: The Australian OCDQ: a decade late, *Journal of Educational Administration* 23, 53-58, 1985.
13. Brooke Army Medical Center: Mission statement, San Antonio, Tex. http://www.gprmc.amedd.army.mil/ (Retrieved February 8, 2007.)
14. Borkowski N: *Organizational behavior in health care*, Sudbury, Mass., 2005, Jones and Bartlett.
15. Burns JM: *Leadership*, New York, 1978, Harper & Row.
16. Cherrington DJ: *The management of human resources,* ed 4, Englewood Cliffs, N.J., 1995, Prentice Hall.
17. Collins J: *Good to great*, New York, 2001, HarperCollins.
18. The Drug-Free Workplace Act of 1988, 41 United States Code Section 701-707.
19. The Drug-Free Workplace Act of 1988, 41 United States Code Section 701(a)(1)(A).
20. Fiedler FE: *A theory of leadership effectiveness*, New York, 1967, McGraw-Hill.
21. French JRP, Raven BH: Bases of social power. In Cartwright D, Zander A (editors): *Group dynamics: research and theory*, New York, 1968, Harper & Row.
22. Gandy J: *Strategic planning: an easy guide*, Alexandria, Va., 2005, American Physical Therapy Association.
23. Gardner J: *On leadership*, New York, 1989, Free Press.
24. Goffee R, Jones G: Why should anyone be led by you? *Harvard Business Review*, pp. 63-70, Sept-Oct 2000.
25. Graen GB, Cashman JF: A role making model in formal organizations: a developmental approach. In Hunt JG, Larson LL (editors): *Leadership frontiers*, Kent, Ohio, 1975, Kent State University Press.
26. Graen GB, Uhl Bien M: The transformation of professionals into self-managing and partially self-designing contributors: towards a theory of leadership making, *Journal of Management Systems* 3: 33-48, 1991.
27. Grant R: *Contemporary strategy analysis: concepts, techniques, and application* (ed 4), Malden, Mass., 2002, Blackwell.
28. Hersey P, Blanchard K: *Management of organizational behavior*, Upper Saddle River, N.J., 1988, Prentice Hall.
29. Herzberg F: *Work and the nature of man*, New York, 1966, The World Publishing Company.
30. House R: A path-goal theory of leader effectiveness, *Administrative Science Quarterly* 16: 321-339, 1971.
31. House RJ, Mitchell TR: Path-goal theory of leadership, *Journal of Contemporary Business* 3(4): 81-87, Autumn 1974.
32. Isaacson N, Ford PJ: Leadership, accountability, and wellness in Organizations, *Journal of Physical Therapy Education* 12(3): 31-38, 1998.
33. Kouzes J, Posner B: *The leadership challenge*, San Francisco, 2002, Jossey Bass.
34. Kraemer TJ: Leaders and leadership development: Part II, *The Resource: Newsletter of the Section on Administration/APTA* 30(4): 1, 4-12, 2000.
35. Kraybill R: Style matters: The Kraybill Conflict Style Inventory, Riverhouse ePress. http://www.riverhouseepress.com/Conflict_Style_Inventory.htm. (Retrieved August 10, 2006.)
36. Lewin K, Llippit R, White R: Patterns of aggressive behavior in experimentally created social climates, *Journal of Social Psychology* 10: 271-301, 1939.
37. Likert R: *The human organization: its management and value*, New York, 1967, McGraw-Hill.

38. Maslow AH: *Motivation and personality,* New York, 1954, Harper Row.
39. *Merriam-Webster's Collegiate Dictionary* (ed 11), Springfield, Mass., 2004, Merriam-Webster.
40. Noble DF: *America by design: science, technology, and the rise of corporate capitalism,* New York, 1977, Knopf.
41. Porter M: *Competitive strategy: techniques for analyzing industries and competitors,* New York, 1998, Free Press.
42. Prochaska PO, DiClemente CC: Transtheoretical therapy: toward a more integrative model of change, *Psychotherapy: Theory, Research and Practice* 19: 276-278, 1982.
43. Rooke D, Torbert W: Seven transformations of leadership, *Harvard Business Review* 67-76, April, 2005.
44. Scott RW: Defending the apparently indefensible urinalysis client in nonjudicial proceedings, *Army Lawyer* 55-60, November 1986.

45. Scott RW: *Promoting legal awareness in physical and occupational therapy*, St. Louis, 1997, Mosby.
46. Tannenbaum R, Schmidt W: How to choose a leadership pattern, *Harvard Business Review* 51(3): 1-10, 1973.
47. Thomas K: Conflict and negotiation processes in organizations. In Dunnette M (editor): *Handbook of industrial and organizational psychology* (ed 2, vol 3), Palo Alto, Calif., 1992, Consulting Psychologists Press.
48. Thomas K, Kilmann R: Thomas-Kilmann Conflict Mode Instrument, Tuxedo, N.Y., 1974, Xicom (currently available through Consulting Psychologist Press).
49. Vroom V, Yetton P: *Leadership and decision-making*, Pittsburgh, 1973, University of Pittsburgh Press.

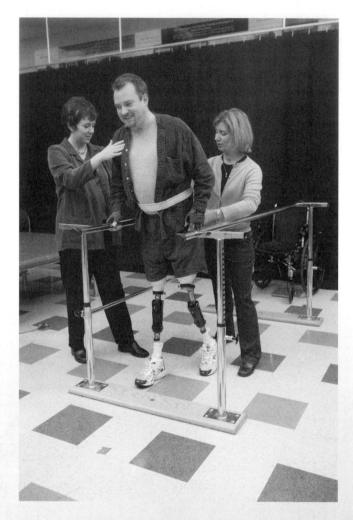

Courtesy University of Indianapolis.

Human Resource Management in Physical Therapy Settings

Ron Scott

ABSTRACT

One of the key aspects of physical therapy clinical leadership is the management of human resources, which facilitates effective clinical operations. From recruitment and selection to retention and professional development, the management of human resources is both time intensive and critically important to the success of the practice. This chapter explores these topics, as well as employee performance appraisal, discipline, compensation management, and labor-management relations. Selected case presentations and exercises are interspersed throughout the chapter.

KEY WORDS AND PHRASES

Behaviorally anchored
  rating scale
Benefits
Compensation management
Contractors
Counseling
Covenants
Covenant not to compete
Discipline
Dismissal
Employee assistance
  program
Ethics
Forced-choice appraisal
  rating instrument

Forecasting
Graphic rating scale
Human relations movement
Human resource
  management
Incentives
Interviews
Job sharing
Labor
Management by exception
  (MBE)
Management by
  objectives (MBO)
Management-labor relations
Markov analysis

Nonsolicitation clause
Paid time off (PTO)
Performance appraisal
Personnel management
Progressive discipline
Recruitment
Retention
Scientific management
Time-and-motion studies
Union representative
Weingarten rule
Work-life balance

1. Understand the importance of human resource inputs to successful business operations, and value them accordingly.

2. Define the seven classic human resource management functions, and relate them to physical therapy business management in clinical and educational settings.

3. Apply chapter principles to human resource recruitment, selection, and retention in clinical and other physical therapy practice settings.

4. In cooperation with co-professionals, develop optimal performance appraisal systems and instruments for specific physical therapy business environments.

5. Evaluate the systems approach to employee training, education, and development, and, if effective, implement it in practice.

6. Describe total compensation and its relation to employee growth, loyalty, productivity, and satisfaction.

7. Devise, disseminate, and implement a continuum of employee discipline tools using the constructive or rehabilitative approach.

8. Educate employees in physical therapy settings about employee assistance programs, and encourage their judicious use.

9. Seriously, fairly, and thoroughly evaluate all employee grievances, and take appropriate resolute action in response to them.

10. Effectively manage and foster the professional development of an increasingly diverse workforce.

INTRODUCTION: THE IMPORTANCE OF HUMAN RESOURCE MANAGEMENT

No aspect of business management is more critically important than the effective management of human resources, or people working within a business organization or system. Human inputs drive business operations, promote productivity, and directly and intimately control the bottom line, whether an enterprise is operated for-profit (i.e., business owners and/or shareholders realize a net monetary gain [or loss] from operations) or not-for-profit (i.e., non-distributable net operating revenue results from business operations).

Business managers at all levels have always known these facts or truisms, yet until relatively recently, **human resource management** was not officially recognized as a professional endeavor. Now, in virtually every professional and graduate business education program (including health professional entry-level and postprofessional education programs), students undertake formal required and elective coursework in human resource management so that they may effectively and optimally manage workforces once they are in the field or in practice.

HUMAN RESOURCE VERSUS PERSONNEL MANAGEMENT

Human resource management differs greatly from **personnel management** in philosophy and application. While the latter is concerned principally with maximization of production or service outputs, the former addresses the individual and collective needs of the human inputs that produce those outputs.[23] Human resource management is, as a philosophical approach, of relative recent vintage.[58]

Personnel Management

Personnel management is a traditional term that refers to management of people resources. It was developed during the Industrial Revolution to describe the physical management of industrial workers. As a management approach, personnel management is relatively bureaucratic in nature—closed to outside influences and rigid in its policies and procedures. It is focused on process and output. Systematically, it is reactive, rather than proactive, in the face of workplace problems, issues, and dilemmas.

In terms of performance assessment, personnel management focuses on compliance by employees with minimally acceptable workplace standards. Within this system, performance expectations of employees are typically well-defined and well-understood. For example, one standard might require a hospital-based staff physical therapist to interact with two patients per hour for 8 consecutive hours per workday.

Scientific management is characteristic of industry-based personnel management, such as exists in auto- or steel-production facilities. Frederick W. Taylor is known as the father of scientific management, within which the optimal processes of job performance are delineated by experts or by consensus (of management), and workers are trained to carry out those work tasks but given little or no say in their development or modification.

Taylor advocated employee compensation exclusively on the basis of the objectively determined complexity of the work to be performed. According to this philosophy, the more complex a given task is, the higher is the rate of employee compensation. Taylor also advocated piece-rate incentive compensation, under which workers are rewarded according to the quantity of work product produced in an hour, day, or other pay period. The modern-day manifestation of this philosophy is the concept of "billable hours."

Two of Taylor's protégées were Lillian and Frank Gilbreth. The Gilbreths are best known for developing specialized processes for assessing quantitative and qualitative aspects of industrial employees' workplace performance through **time-and-motion studies**. In time-and-motion studies, supervisors observe employee performance of duties over a given time period and analyze processes, count outputs, or both.

Time-and-motion studies are still common today, and their use has expanded beyond industrial workplace settings into, for example, clinical health care delivery settings, such as physical therapy clinical and home health practices. As part of utilization review or other quality management measures, professional colleagues may observe physical therapists, assistants, and extenders in the performance of cognitive (examination, evaluation, diagnosis, and prognosis), psychomotor (interventional), and affective (interactional) aspects of clinical practice.

Physical therapy and other primary health professionals may react adversely to direct observation of their professional patient care activities for purposes of employee **performance appraisal**. In lieu of direct observation, a self-directed time-and-motion study can be used instead, in which health professional employees generate their own running logs of daily workplace activities (for a reasonable period of time, such as 1 or 2 days) on the honor system. Managers can then review the logs, after submission, for compliance with quantitative productivity standards.

Regarding quantitative productivity standards for physical therapy professionals in general, these standards must be reasonable. The practice of clinical physical therapy is among the most physically and mentally demanding and time-intensive disciplines, similar in nature to clinical nursing, medicine, and surgery. Although the highest qualitative productivity standards should be expected of every employee in every work setting, quantitative productivity standards must be evidence based, derived from published norms established by input from physical therapist and public health experts and by consensus among clinical managers and working-level professionals.

Human Resource Management

The philosophy of human resource management began in the 1920s, during which time Dr. Elton Mayo of Harvard University began to carry out qualitative research involving employee motivation, performance, and group dynamics. Mayo's famous studies were known as the Hawthorne studies because they were carried out at the Hawthorne Works of Western Electric, in Cicero, Illinois.

Mayo assessed the many variegated elements of telephone–assembly-line work, such as lighting conditions, piece-rate incentive compensation, workstation design, and work-group dynamics. He concluded that, more than monetary **incentives**, amicable supervision and self-determination over work processes and quality of workmanship resulted in greater workplace productivity.

Mayo's conclusions led to the development of the term **human relations movement** as a branch of people management. This philosophy of people management focuses on people as essential, indispensable inputs of ultimate value, responsible for the generation of commercial products and services, not merely as inanimate inputs of production, as is the case under scientific management.[32]

World War II brought additional changes to the way in which workers are managed and led in the workplace. At the advent of World War II, millions of civilians in the United States had to be rapidly inducted into military service. Their cognitive abilities, psychomotor skills, interests, and affect had to be assessed in relatively short order so as to assign the new soldiers to positions that would lead to victory in the war. As part of that effort, abilities and interest inventories and related instruments were devised and implemented, and close attention was paid to service member morale, which, it came to be realized, directly influenced productivity and the outcome of the war.

The profession of human resource management developed as a direct result of World War II. From the end of World War II until today, the human relations model has predominated as the gold standard for people management.

It is a truism that workers, especially physical therapy professionals, are complex human beings with complex needs and wants. Human resource managers address, with sensitivity to employee privacy concerns, personal and familial interests, including, among myriad other areas, continuing education, training, and development; improved patient care delivery processes; enhanced **benefits** and incentives for high-quality work; optimal, safe working conditions; multicultural interpersonal interaction[54]; travel and consultation opportunities; organizational recognition for excellent service; retirement security and comfort; and health care (including dental, mental health, and vision care services) and legal benefits. In a managed care era in which cost-containment–focused organizational interests predominate, the human resource manager faces the herculean task of supplying enough of these employee and family demand inputs to keep employees satisfied and motivated,[15,16,37] so as to comply with the organization's social responsibility owed to its workforce and to society.[61]

Classic Human Resource Management Functions

Cherrington[12] classified the functional roles of human resource managers and their staffs into seven classes of activities, which are as applicable to physical therapy clinical settings as they are to every other business organization (Box 2-1).

The first of these human resource management responsibilities encompasses the global concept of employment. Employment encompasses the complete range of staffing issues, including **forecasting** future worker needs and qualifications, **recruitment** and selection processes, and **retention** of the workforce. Performance and competency assessment activities help ensure state-of-the-art patient care

---

BOX **2-1** ■ **Classic Human Resource Management Functional Roles**

1. Employment: forecasting, recruitment, selection, and retention
2. Performance/competency assessment of employees, contractors, and relevant others
3. Compensation management
4. Training, education, and development of workers
5. Maintenance of management-employee relations; coordination of grievance and discipline procedures
6. Management of organization health, safety, and wellness programs
7. Human research management research activities

delivery and appropriate, focused professional development of staff. **Compensation management** involves management of all three aspects of employee compensation: salary/wages, benefits (including deferred retirement benefits), and incentives. Training, education, and employee development entails production and delivery of individual and group instruction across the spectrum of appropriate experiences, from safety and health education to professional development to formal continuing education. Human resource managers also participate proactively in **management-labor relations**, whether in unionized or nonunionized environments. They also are responsible for management of organizational safety, health, and prevention/wellness programs and initiatives,[7,59] including community outreach activities and events such as health fairs. Finally, like all professionals, human resource management professionals must conduct discipline-specific, evidence-based research to justify their activities, budgets, and proposals.

These employment-related issues are especially important to managers of physical therapy services. For most of the second half of the twentieth century and the beginning of the twenty-first century, aggregate demand for physical therapy professional services has far exceeded the available supply of physical therapy professionals in the marketplace. The marketing adage that has traditionally attracted many college students to seek out physical therapy as a career is "ten jobs for every graduate." In addition to expected job security, students normally choose to join the physical therapy discipline for altruistic and human service reasons.

The scarcity of the human resources supply of available physical therapists led to the design and employment of creative solutions to ameliorate shortages. Incentives included, among others, lucrative sign-on and retention money bonuses, generous continuing education benefits (including subsidies for advanced degree study), and **paid time off (PTO)** for research and other professional development activities.

Factors such as increased competition from other health care providers, managed care health services delivery, and restrictive federal and other third-party payer (TTP) reimbursement policies have some dampening effect on the need for or utilization of physical therapy professionals.[66]

STAFFING ISSUES

The ability to meet patient demand needs—often in multiple care centers—requires careful attention by clinical and human resource managers to key professional and support staffing.[21] Clinical health professional and support staffing is often a careful balance of utilization of employees, **contractors**, volunteers, and others.

Forecasting Employment Needs

It is critical for business operations to have an adequate number of employees in place to satisfy consumer demand and needs. Nowhere is this truism more fundamental than in clinical health care service delivery, where patient well-being literally depends on the presence and intervention of competent professional and support staff.

To accurately assess the demand for new employees, clinical and human resource managers employ both qualitative and quantitative processes. One commonly used quantitative method used by human resource managers for employee forecasting is **Markov analysis**. Markov analysis is a method of probabilistic forecasting in which historical employment data on employee transition between and among various job positions are used to predict current and (immediate) future needs. The following exercise illustrates this simple-to-apply principle.

EXERCISE **2-1**

ABC Medical Center, a level 1 multistate trauma center, provides burn care services to a 10-million-person catchment area population from four states. Historically, the physical therapy services director (whose department staff physical therapists serve as primary burn care specialists for the system) has had difficulty predicting the need for physical therapist burn specialists to staff the burn center in this high turnover environment. The high turnover is largely attributed to burnout from the intense nature of the work. Employment data for the past 5 years (obtained from the center's human resource management research division) are as follows:

Year	PT Staff	Turnover (number of PT staff leaving)	New Hires
2001	3	2	1
2002	2	1	2
2003	3	2	2
2004	3	1	1
2005	3	2	3
2006	4	-	-

What are the expected turnover rates and replacement needs for the burn center (assuming a desired professional staff size of four in the current year)?

DISCUSSION OF EXERCISE 2-1

On the basis of 5-year historical data, the average turnover rate is 57% of professional staff (8 physical therapists out of the 14 employed left their positions). The clinical manager should therefore expect that as many as half of the physical therapist staff may leave by the current year's end and that additional physical therapist-burn specialists must be hired to replace them. The Markov transitional matrix is useful for predicting and justifying additional employee positions, but it does not address the causes of turnover or methods for remediation of the problem.

Recruiting New Employees

Recruitment of new employees[64] in physical therapy, as in all other settings, takes place systematically and in accordance with customary recruitment practices and governing federal, state, and local employment laws and regulations (Box 2-2).

BOX **2-2** ■ **Sequential Steps in the Employee Recruitment Process up to Selection**

1. Forecasting employment needs
2. Organizational authorization for a position
3. Departmental development of a recruitment plan and strategies
4. Development of a position announcement (in coordination with organizational human resources management consultants)
5. Departmental, administrative, and legal review of the position announcement
6. Advertising for the position, including the following:
   a. Internal posting, if appropriate
   b. External dissemination of the position announcement
7. Receipt, screening, and processing of applications for employment
8. Invitations to selected applicants to visit and interview with the organization

Recruitment of new hires may occur from within ("hiring from within") or from sources external to the organization, such as professional education programs.

What are the relative advantages and disadvantages in recruiting from within (i.e., among existing employees) as opposed to recruiting externally for new hires? Possible advantages for recruiting for new positions among current staff include the institutional memory and knowledge of operations, procedures, policies, and formal and informal communication networks among employees within the organization. Also, current employees have a track record of known performance appraisals and are well-known to decision makers within the organization. Finally, organizational employee morale may be enhanced by hiring for new positions among existing staff.

There also may be disadvantages in hiring for new positions among existing staff. Current employees may not offer new creative solutions to current problems as readily as hires from outside the organization. Outside hires may also bring to the organization different practice and educational approaches to physical therapy based on their geographical region of employment and educational experiences.

Alternatives to hiring new employees include such measures as voluntary and mandatory overtime, hiring contract professional and support staff,[50] and mission realignment through compression. Each of these options carries with it relative risks and benefits. Overtime work must comply with federal, state, and local laws and regulations governing its use. Overuse of overtime may adversely affect employee morale and patient safety. Use of contract staff entails greater cost outlays and diminished control of contract staff work product. Mission (professional services) compression may adversely affect a clinic's and organization's bottom line and the community goodwill engendered through service projects.[42,47]

Assuming there are multiple applicants for a given professional position, how many of them should be brought in for an interview, considering how expensive that process can be? Yield ratios often help determine relative numbers in such cases. A yield ratio, like Markov analysis, is a quantitative tool for assessing numbers of job applicants between and among successive recruitment processes on the basis of historical data. Consider the following example:

EXERCISE 2-2

Five-year historical data of XYZ Rehab System shows that for every staff physical therapist position filled, an average of 14 invitations to interview are made, 8 of which are actually carried out. How many invitations and interviews should be anticipated to fill three current staff physical therapist vacancies within the system?

DISCUSSION OF EXERCISE 2-2

# Positions (n)	# Invitations to Interview (nx14)	# Interviews (nx8)
3	42	24

The same equal employment opportunity legal and ethical considerations that govern employment discrimination generally apply to employee recruitment and selection procedures in both the public and private sectors. Job applicants, just like current employees, are protected from employment discrimination by federal statutes, including Title VII of the Civil Rights Act of 1964[13] (which prohibits employment discrimination based on ethnicity, gender,[8,52,65] national origin, race, and religion); the Equal Pay Act of 1963[20] (which requires equal pay for women and men carrying out similar work); the Age Discrimination in Employment Act of 1967[1] (which protects workers and applicants age 40 or older from employment discrimination); and the Americans with Disabilities Act of 1990[3] (which protects physically and mentally disabled workers, job applicants, and those associated with them from employment discrimination), among other statutes, regulations, and case law pronouncements. Of current interest because of the ongoing military conflicts in Afghanistan and Iraq, activated military reservists and National Guard members enjoy job protection under 38 United States Code 2021(b)(3) during periods of activation. Federal, state, and municipal constitutional, case law, and regulatory protection may augment federal statutory protections.

Administrative guidelines promulgated by the Equal Employment Opportunity Commission (EEOC) offer employers specific guidance concerning prohibited and precautionary pre-employment inquiries and information, whether on job applications, in **interviews**, in resumes, or otherwise (Box 2-3).

Precautionary inquiries (i.e., questions that must pass the threshold test of being specifically job-related in order to be legitimate) are also cautioned against (Box 2-4).

BOX **2-3** ▪ **Prohibited Inquiries of Job Candidates**

- Race, ethnicity, national origin (Remember, however, that every employer has the right and legal duty to inquire about any applicant's legal right to work in the United States. This must be carried out universally by prospective employers.)
- Marital status, number of children or other dependents, child care arrangements, existence of an opposite- or same-gender domestic partner
- Religious beliefs or practices
- Disabilities
- Age

BOX **2-4** ▪ **Inquiries of Job Candidates That Are Deemed Precautionary**

- Height or weight
- Education level
- Criminal history (including not only convictions but also arrests)
- Military discharge classification
- Financial status

Most or all of the precautionary inquiries listed in Box 2-4 have been found, in federal administrative and judicial cases, to have had an unfair disparate impact on federally protected classes of people, such as racial and ethnic minorities. Employers may legally inquire about the existence of any applicant's criminal convictions but should include a disclaimer in the job application that an affirmative response will not necessarily preclude selection of the applicant. Instead, indicate that a conviction will be considered in light of the totality of circumstances, including the nature of the offense, the applicant's age at the time the offense occurred, and indices of postconviction rehabilitation. Some of the prohibited and precautionary pre-employment inquiries listed above become legitimate areas for inquiry once an applicant is actually selected for employment (e.g., for benefits activation, EEOC demographics reporting, and other legitimate business and legal needs).

The same considerations apply to résumés.[31,56] Employers are not legally allowed to consider prohibited information in hiring and must exercise special caution when assessing precautionary information (as previously discussed) about prospective employees. As a matter of customary practice, human resource management specialists (and physical therapy clinical managers carrying out human resource management functions in smaller practices without human resource management specialists) typically discard résumés not compliant with legal mandates and precautions.[51,62] Sample résumés with errors present and deleted are shown in Exercise 2-3.

EXERCISE 2-3

The following resume contains at least 10 errors. Spot and highlight them.

Paul Joplin, DPT
470 Bending Tree
San Antono, Texas 78200

Home: 210-555-1213
Cell: 210-555-1214
Email: pj@anywhere.net

Marital Status: Married, 2 chilren
Permanent U.S. Residant
Date of Birth: Dec. 19, 1851

Religion: Methodist
National Origin: Iran
Height: 68 inches,
Weight: 280 pounds

Objective: To continue to utilize my best clinical judgment and skills to effect optimal therapeutic results for my patients in a dynamic outpatient orthopedic physical therapy practice.

| Experience: | *2004-present* | ABC medical Center, Ortho Clinic Director |
| | | Universal City, TX   210-555-1215 |

Led team of 5 professionals in caring for geriatric patients with orthopedic conditions.

| | *2002-2004* | Koby School District, Physical Therapist |
| | Judson ISD | Universal City, TX   210-555-1216 |

Consulted for IEP teams for students with disabilities.
Developed new protocol for standing table for students.

| | *2000-2002* | Missionary, United Methodist Church |
| | | Zimbabwe, Africa |

	1999-2000	Medical Clerk, Drs. Smith and Jones, P.C.
		Performed a widely variegated range of
		administrative tasks.

Education:	*1994-1999*	XYZ DPT Program
		Anytown, USA
		Dean's List

| Avocations: | Conversational in Spanish; enjoy international travel and playing guitar |

| References: | Available upon request |

Sample Physical Therapist Résumé for Management Review (Errors Corrected)

Paul Joplin, DPT
470 Bending Tree   Home: 210-555-1213
San Antonio, Texas 78200   Cell: 210-555-1214
                                                    Email: pj@anywhere.net

Objective: To continue to utilize my best clinical judgment and skills to effect optimal
therapeutic results for my patients in a dynamic outpatient orthopedic physical
therapy practice.

Experience:	*2004-present*	ABC Medical Center, Ortho Clinic Director
		Universal City, TX 210-555-1215

Led team of 5 professionals in caring for geriatric patients
with orthopedic conditions. Led JCAHO rehab survey team
to commendation in August 2005 survey.

	2002-2004	Koby School District, Physical Therapist
	Judson ISD	Universal City, TX 210-555-1216

Consulted for IEP teams for students with disabilities.
Developed new protocol for standing table for students.

	2000-2002	Missionary, United Methodist Church
		Zimbabwe, Africa
	1999-2000	Medical Clerk, Drs. Smith and Jones, P.C.
		Performed a widely variegated range of
		administrative tasks.
Education:	*1994-1999*	XYZ DPT Program
		Anytown, USA
		Dean's List
Avocations:	Conversational in Spanish; enjoy international travel and playing guitar	
References:	Available upon request	

What are the purposes and formats for applicant interviews? The principal
purpose for a pre-employment interview is to interact with the prospective
employee in person and obtain job-relevant information from him or her.[26,63] The
pre-employment interview also provides an excellent opportunity for the
organization to showcase itself and establish initial rapport with a prospective
employee.[11,53] Be aware, though, that first impressions may not always reflect the

true character of either a job applicant or an employing organization. Additional in-person visits and interviews should be considered before offers of employment are extended or accepted.

Interview formats include structured, semistructured, and unstructured interviews.[33] In structured interviews, interviewers (alone or in groups) ask precisely the same questions to all interviewees. The key advantages of such interviews include due process, or fundamental fairness, to interviewees and uniformity of applicant inputs for employers. The structured interview is obviously the most reliable (repeatable) of the interview types, regardless of whether the same interviewer conducts the interviews for a given position. Semistructured interviews involve augmenting structured questions with supplemental applicant- or circumstance-specific additional questions. Unstructured or nondirective interviews contain general, open-ended questions, which allow the interviewee to set the course of its content. The unstructured interview is the most unreliable (unpredictable) interview type.

Under its four-fifths rule, the federal Equal Employment Opportunity Commission attributes as possible evidence of disparate discriminatory impact in applicant selection employee selection rates for protected classes that are less than four fifths or 80% of the rate of selection for nonprotected-class job applicants. The following example illustrates this principle:

EXERCISE 2-4

Thirty applicants are hired as home health aides for a new managed care organization (MCO). Forty Caucasian males applied for the positions, as did 40 females (30 Caucasians and 10 African-Americans). Among the successful applicants are 20 white men and 10 women (7 Caucasian, 3 African-American). Has the EEOC's four-fifths rule been violated?

DISCUSSION OF EXERCISE 2-4

Yes. The selection rate for white males was 50%. To avoid closer EEOC scrutiny, the selection rate for women should have been at least 40% (80% of 50%). In this case, only 25% of women applicants (10 of 40 women) were selected for employment.

Negligent Hiring/Retention Liability

Employers, especially in hands-on clinical health care disciplines such as physical therapy, must be cognizant of potential liability exposure for negligent hiring of dangerous employees who may injure patients, clients, staff, or others.[14] Negligent hiring liability arises whenever an employer fails to take reasonable steps before the new employee is hired to investigate that employee's background (e.g., through licensing board and public records reviews). Employers in physical therapy clinical settings should take appropriate steps to screen all applicants for potential dangerousness through pre-employment inquiries about criminal convictions and gaps in employment and in education and by conducting appropriate background investigations (such as screening public records for convictions), pursuant to signed releases by applicants.

Background investigations for licensed professionals must include queries to the federal National Practitioner Data Bank (www.npdb-hipdb.hrsa.gov/npdb) concerning adverse credentialing, licensing and privileging actions, and malpractice payments in settlement or judgment. In addition, employers should physically check with as many résumé references as is feasible and document and securely retain reference responses.

Restrictive Covenants in Employment Contracts

Restrictive covenants in employment contracts limit the ability of parties to act without legal restraint in specified ways.[69] In health care employment contracts specifically, the principal types of restrictive covenants include nonsolicitation contractual clauses and **covenants** (or contractual promises) not to compete.[71] A **nonsolicitation clause** in an employment contract prevents a former professional employee from marketing his or her professional services to the former employer's existing clientele. A **covenant not to compete** prevents a former employee from competing directly (normally in a finite geographic market, although subject to change with the growth of web-based businesses) with the former employer for a specified period of time.

A covenant not to compete is, in essence, an agreed-to restraint of trade, which is generally considered by the law to be against public policy as an antitrust violation (Box 2-5). For that reason, some state laws disallow them altogether.[41] Most states do permit them, however, as a means to protect legitimate employer interests.[70]

Health Professional Student Pre-employment Contracts

The successful negotiation of pre-employment contracts permits many health professional students to contribute meaningfully toward self-funding of their professional education, without being saddled with enormous loan debt upon entering the workforce. Employers also benefit from pre-employment contracting

---

BOX **2-5** ▪ **General Required Elements of a Valid Covenant not to Compete**

- Consideration: written contractual evidence that an employee's promise not to compete with the employer after employment is bargained for and supported by reciprocal value
- Reasonableness in terms of geographic scope of coverage, specific practice restrictions, and specific time frames for enforcement

with health professional students in that staffing processes are made more predictable, with relatively firm work commitments on the part of scarce prospective health care professionals.

There are, however, several important potential disadvantages to pre-employment contracting. The process of seeking out and negotiating pre-employment contracts may foster excessive competition among students in selected job markets and practice settings. Employment contracts are formal legal instruments just like any other business contract with legal and ethical obligations incumbent upon both parties, including penalties for breaches of respective promises. Such contracts are often very complex, containing elements such as conditions precedent to the receipt of any employment bonuses and liquidated (pre-agreed) monetary damages provisions for nonperformance. There are also tax consequences for students who receive monetary payments from current or future employers. All parties to such agreements should have them reviewed by their respective legal counsel before signing them.

Students also need to be cognizant of potential ethical dilemmas associated with pre-employment agreements. Potential issues include the hypothetical student who shops for alternative employment after having already signed a contractual pre-employment agreement with another entity from whom the student may have received monies. Also, students under contract may be the subject of an actual or perceived conflict of interest for alleged preferential treatment while they are on clinical affiliations, compared with their colleagues not under contract. The American Physical Therapy Association (APTA) has developed guidelines for student pre-employment contracting, which should be reviewed by employers, students, and educators before such agreements are reached.

EMPLOYEE RETENTION ISSUES

Employee selection is one side of the professional staffing coin. Retention of key employees is the other. What incentives are required to keep physical therapy professionals in a given work setting?

A principal monetary incentive for professional employee retention in physical therapy is the retention bonus (analogous to the sign-on bonus for recruitment). Nonmonetary incentives to professional employee retention may be more important than monetary ones. Schein assembled a list of career anchors comprising perceived career attributes deemed important to professionals. They include job security,[48] autonomy over one's work product (i.e., professional autonomy), competence enhancements (including continuing education, training, and development), and the ability to be or become more creative and inventive on the job.[2,40,43,45,46]

Other nonmonetary employee retention incentives focus on fostering employees' **work-life balance.**[49] These include, among others, **job sharing**, job redesign, compressed work schedules, and appropriate accommodation of employees' religious beliefs and practices, illnesses, and grief over the loss of a loved one.

According to Vedantam, technological advancements makes it easy for employers to exploit professional employees by requiring them to respond to email and cell phone inquiries around the clock.[68] Vedantam also noted that one in six married couples seeks a situation in which both partners work part-time. Currently, though, only one in 50 couples achieves this goal.

Incentives to employee retention have legal as well as professional dimensions. Digh[17] suggested that employers ask themselves the following questions related to employee religious accommodation[17]:

1. What, if any, are the noncost reasons to grant or deny the accommodation?
2. What is the organization's history concerning granting religious accommodation requests?
3. Has the employee offered any potential compromises?

Letters of Recommendation: To Write or Not to Write?

Employers, professors, clinical educators, managers, and other professionals are frequently asked to write letters of recommendation for employees, students, volunteers, and others. Prospective writers of such letters of recommendation may be ethically torn between the conflicting interests of helping someone whom they may like personally and conveying accurate information about the person. Many human resource managers believe that letters of recommendation may be of little value because of inherent bias. Cherrington reported that employers typically disregard them unless they contain negative information.[12]

Writers of letters of recommendation are often constrained from making candid comments about a candidate because of the fear of exposure to liability. The legal morass surrounding letters of recommendation is indeed complex. Potential liability over letters of recommendation may be based on the following:

1. Defamation of character (i.e., the communication of false information that is injurious to a person's positive reputation in the geographic and professional community). Slander is defamation communicated orally, whereas libel is defamation communicated in other, more permanent forms, such as in writing or on audiotape or videotape.
2. Invasion of privacy—specifically, the public disclosure of private facts about an employee or job applicant, including information about criminal background, drug use, HIV status, and sexual orientation. Courts have found liable, and have imposed punitive damages against, business organizations that unlawfully release such private information about employees or former employees.
3. Intentional infliction of emotional distress—that is, unreasonable and outrageous conduct (potentially including the dissemination of sensitive personal information about an employee or former employee) that results in severe physical and emotional injury to the victim.

At the opposite end of the legal spectrum, individuals may also face liability exposure for failing to provide an accurate reference when they have agreed (or are otherwise bound) to do so, as when such a duty is delineated in an

---

BOX 2-6 ■ Reducing Litigation Risks Associated With Recommendation Letters

1. Require a written request for information from a prospective employer or other requestor rather than accepting such a request by telephone or email.
2. Require a written release from a candidate (especially when a recommendation might be less than stellar) before releasing any information about him or her.
3. Respond to request for information about current or former employees only in writing so that your words cannot be misconstrued. Maintain file copies of such correspondence for at least the period of the legal statute of limitations (deadline for bringing a lawsuit). Check with legal counsel for this state-specific time period and related advice.
4. If possible, centralize responses to recommendation and reference requests. Have the organization's human resource manager or legal advisor (or both) review and then send out all responses to requests for such information.

---

employee handbook or employment contract. Litigation based on discrimination might also result if one candidate learns that an employer or other official has written a favorable recommendation for one colleague but has refused to do so for the litigant.

The ongoing concern over potential litigation involving letters of recommendation has caused many, if not most, employers to change their previous liberal policies regarding writing them. Many employers limit the information they are willing to convey to basic employment data such as inclusive dates of employment and positions held. This self-limitation applies even though writers of letters of recommendation enjoy qualified immunity in many states, as long as they report their opinions in good faith.

As rehabilitation helping professionals, physical therapist clinicians, educators, and managers usually want to be helpful to former employees seeking references for employment or education (Box 2-6).

Performance Appraisal

Employee performance appraisals are important critical pathways for key human resource–related employee actions, from pay adjustments to training and development to discipline and even discharge from employment. This is true across all business organizations, irrespective of size, and especially true of physical therapy practices, in which employee interests are of crucial concern to management.

There is no legal requirement that any business organization have in place an employee performance appraisal system. Civil rights laws do require, however, that systems in use be fair and applied across organizations or systems (i.e., from top to bottom). Similarly, employee performance appraisal systems must conform to applicable ethical standards, especially APTA's *Code of Ethics* and *Implementing Guide for Professional Conduct*.

EXERCISE 2-5

As an individual or group exercise, peruse the American Physical Therapy Association's *Code of Ethics* and *Implementing Guide for Professional Conduct,* and annotate which provisions might apply, directly or indirectly, to performance appraisal systems and processes. If you are completing the exercise in groups, share results within and among small groups.

When establishing performance appraisal systems, physical therapy managers must ascertain what precise employee attributes are to be evaluated.[22] Are personalities being judged? If so, what justification exists for their appraisal? Are employee behaviors being assessed? If so, to what end? What are most likely being assessed from employees' efforts are outcomes and outputs. Attempting to assess employee personalities or behaviors may engender ethical, legal, and relevancy issues.

As managers, when assessing employees be sure to minimize use of the halo (perfection personified) effect for individual employees. Most workers are good employees who deserve fair, accurate, and objectively good performance ratings. To assess everyone as superlative invalidates the process by failing to provide accurate feedback to employees and to the organization. Similarly, raters should avoid using the central tendency effect, or averaging of employees under performance appraisal systems, which unfairly deflates truly superlative employee performance by dampening rating inflation.

Performance Appraisal Tools

The types of performance evaluation instruments vary widely. Four main typologies predominate, however. The simplest and least effective (because it fails to adequately describe performance) of these is the forced-choice employee performance appraisal instrument, in which standardized, pre-established word or phrase descriptors are selected by evaluators rating employees. Figure 2-1 illustrates an example of a **forced-choice appraisal rating instrument**.

Rate this physical therapist's overall performance this rating period by checking the appropriate entry:	
Always exceeds performance objectives	_____
Usually exceeds performance objectives	_____
Sometimes achieves performance objectives	_____
Seldom or never achieves performance objectives	_____

FIGURE 2-1 | Forced choice performance appraisal summary rating.

Professional-patient/client relations. Place an "x" along the continuum for this ratee's professional relations with patients under his or her care.

| Superlative | Good | Needs improvement |

FIGURE 2-2 | Graphic rating scale performance assessment of a physical therapist's professional relations with patients under care.

Another performance appraisal system is the **graphic rating scale**. This performance appraisal instrument is used to assess various aspects of critical job performance and is similar to a visual analog pain scale familiar to all clinical physical therapists.

The APTA Clinical Performance Instrument (CPI) for student affiliates is an example of a graphic rating scale. Another example appears in Figure 2-2, in which a rater assesses physical therapist-patient relations.

Another performance appraisal instrument is the **behaviorally anchored rating scale**, which is similar to the graphic rating scale but includes much more richly annotated performance descriptors. An example appears in Figure 2-3.

Employers, particularly in clinical health care delivery environments, are beginning to use multi-input performance appraisal instruments (e.g., 270/360-degree performance appraisal instruments, which may include input from superiors, peers, subordinates, patients, and relevant others).[70] While such instruments may give decision-makers broader input regarding employee performance, there are pitfalls associated with their use. Confidentiality issues must be considered. Human resource management consultants often recommend redacting names or other personal identifiers of those persons giving input to maximize confidentiality. However, rated employees may challenge such confidentiality measures

Professional-patient/client relations. Place an "x" along the continuum for the ratee's professional relations with patients under his or her care.

Superlative	Good	Needs improvement
Empathetic, excellent history-taking and superlative communication skills.	Sympathetic, good history-taking skills, good communication skills.	Needs to work on bedside manner, history-taking skills, patient/family communications.

FIGURE 2-3 | Behaviorally anchored rating scale performance assessment of a physical therapist's professional relations with patients under care.

(e.g., by asserting that false information was provided by input sources). Another fairness issue involves the propriety of peers assessing one another on performance appraisals. While this is routinely done during peer review as part of quality improvement programs, it may not be appropriate to have employees assess one another during performance appraisal, particularly when limited promotion or pay increase opportunities are available.

EXERCISE 2-6

After organizing into small groups, develop and share sample performance appraisal instruments of various types for selected physical therapy clinical environments and classifications of professionals (e.g., orthopedic outpatient clinic, academic medical center, school-based setting, physical therapists and assistants, and clerical workers).

The Process of Employee Appraisal

What processes are involved in employee performance appraisal? The initial step in employee performance appraisal is to develop a richly annotated job description for each employee undergoing evaluation. Job descriptions should delineate critical and ancillary job functions. What is a core and what is an ancillary job function are case-by-case determinations made by management as a matter of business judgment.[28] The distinction is critically important. Accommodation pursuant to the Americans with Disabilities Act is required, where appropriate, for critical, but not ancillary, job functions for disabled employees and/or job applicants.

The next step in the performance appraisal process is the establishment of employee performance objectives for the given rating period, which should be divided into major and secondary performance objectives. The rater and ratee should meet at the beginning of the rating period and plan to meet periodically at regular intervals (and *ad hoc*, as required) thereafter during the rating period for **counseling** and strategizing. At the end of the rating period, the parties meet formally for the performance appraisal interview, from which a written report is generated.

Peter Drucker (1909-2005), in 1954, developed a superlative performance appraisal system, which has come to be known as **management by objectives (MBO).** MBO is both a management philosophy and a performance appraisal system. It is empowering and proactive and is characterized by shared responsibility over performance appraisal between a rater and rated employee. Under MBO, the rater and rated employee jointly develop and accept responsibility for employee performance objectives, which mesh with the organization's goals and philosophy. The focus of appraisal is on outcomes, not employee behaviors or personalities. Before final evaluation, the rated employee carries out a self-appraisal, which becomes part of the evaluation interview and report. The primary purpose for employee performance appraisal under MBO is always educative and never punitive. **Management by exception (MBE)** is similar to MBO, except that counseling and ratings are based exclusively on conformity or nonconformity with pre-established performance objectives.

   Raters are cautioned, whether employing MBO or another system, to use what Cherrington describes as the "sandwich technique" when making evaluative comments about performance to employee-ratees. This technique requires that positive performance be recognized both before and after critical or negative comments are made.

EMPLOYEE TRAINING, EDUCATION, AND DEVELOPMENT

Employee training, education, and development are related core human resource management functions that are of crucial importance for maintaining employee professional competence, optimizing patient satisfaction with services, and fostering employee self-actualization through professional growth. The processes of developing, delivering, and monitoring efficacy of training, education, and development programs are the joint responsibility of clinical and human resource managers in medium-sized to large organizations.

   Perhaps the most efficient way of managing continuing education, training, and development is through the use of von Bertalanfy's systems model, within which a feedback loop is employed to optimize efficacy and efficiency of effort and expenditures. Under the systems model, managers first evaluate training, education, and development program needs. Next, they develop and prioritize program opportunities, then select one or more of them for adoption. Once implemented, the continuing education, training, and development programs are evaluated on an ongoing basis for efficiency and efficacy. Feedback comes from direct observation, consultant input, pretest and post-test instrument scores, and employee evaluations, among other means. If they meet organizational and employee needs, the programs are retained. If not, modifications or substitutions result, so as to optimize results and validate the expenditure associated with such initiatives. A depiction of the systems approach to employee training, education, and development appears in Figure 2-4.

   Employee training, education, and development may take place on- or off-site, using a wide range of presentation media, from self-study or programmed study to lectures or lab sessions. The appropriateness of the means of instruction depends in large part on the skill set to be developed, be it psychomotor clinical skill

---

Assess employee education, training, and development needs

Evaluate education, training, and development opportunities

Prioritize them and implement the optimal one(s)

Test them for efficacy and effectiveness

Substitute alternative opportunities, as needed

FIGURE 2-4 | Systems modeled for employee continuing education, training, and development activities.

development (e.g., wound debridement) to cognitive skills (e.g., coding for billing for services) to education, training, and development addressing primarily the affective domain (e.g., **ethics** and legal instruction).

Different levels of employees have different, focused training, education, and development needs.[27] For example, managerial professionals and administrators may require more global, conceptual education experiences geared toward relevant cognitive development (e.g., leadership and negotiations courses), whereas clinical physical therapists and assistants may require more psychomotor skill development related to their clinical services delivery (e.g., therapeutic exercise and wound debridement courses). First-line supervisors and middle managers may require a mix of cognitive and psychomotor-focused instruction. Employees at all levels require affective-focused ethical, legal, and interpersonal skills development.

What are the relative advantages and disadvantages of on- and off-site employee training, education, and development? On-site training, education, and development experiences probably entail lower cost, are easier to prepare for and manage, and facilitate easier monitoring of employee attendance and participation. Off-site training, education, and development experiences give employees greater potential opportunities to interact with peers from outside the organization and learn about different work methods and approaches. They also provide an uninterrupted respite from the workplace, giving employees a better chance to concentrate, retain information, and recharge their batteries so that they come back to the organization refreshed and motivated. Consider, though, the following case example:

EXERCISE **2-7**

Three physical therapist-employees of ABC Health Systems—Joe P., Ron Q, and Jonathan X—are sent away to an organization-funded 1-week orthopedic physical therapy mobilization course in Flagstaff, Arizona. Joe attends all sessions and works diligently therein. Ron and Jonathan go off to play in Las Vegas during days 3 through 5 of the course, attending only 4 of 7 days. Upon returning, Joe informs his supervisor, Misty, of Ron and Jon's antics. Misty promises Joe anonymity for reporting his colleagues' suspected misconduct. What should be done?

DISCUSSION OF EXERCISE 2-7

Misty should consult with human resource management for advice. She may wish to have the employees summarize their experiences separately in journals and submit the journals to her for review. She also may solicit feedback from the course instructor regarding the employees' attendance and performance on any pre- and post-tests administered at the course. Misty may also require the employees to make presentations on what they learned at the course within, for example, a 15-day period after returning. It would be difficult for her to confront Ron and Jon because of her promise of confidentiality to Joe. Whatever she elects to do, a policy should be developed and disseminated detailing requirements for attendance and participation for future ABC employees sent to, and funded by, the organization for training, education, and development.

COMPENSATION MANAGEMENT

Another core human resource management role is management of compensation involving employees, contractors, consultants, and relevant others. Total compensation consists of salary (normally reserved exclusively for professional employees) and wages, benefits, and monetary incentives. Employee compensation has multiple co-primary objectives. It serves to motivate employees to continuously improve performance. It is designed to be equitable, internally and externally, so that employees sense that their relative worth is recognized and rewarded. It must be legal and ethical, in conformity with laws such as the Fair Labor Standards Act, which requires the payment of supplemental wages for overtime. Finally, compensation policy must be in keeping with prudent financial management principles.

Organizations must ensure that their established pay levels and ranges match stated job descriptions and are competitive. Competitiveness of compensation in clinical physical therapy practice is a recurrent issue. Although there may be periods of relative stability in employee supply and demand, which consequently stabilizes salaries, wages, and related compensation, the supply of, and demand for, physical therapists and assistants may fluctuate greatly, leading to waxing and waning compensation packages.

Data regarding employee salaries, wages, and related compensation issues are confidential matters. A cardinal rule of business organizations, which should be expressly stated in employee handbooks, is that each employee is prohibited from sharing the details of compensation packages with fellow employees, except where allowed by law. In most business organizations, it is a disciplinary offense to share confidential compensation information with co-workers.

The Equal Pay Act of 1963 mandates equal pay for men and women doing the same or substantially similar work.[20] The Equal Pay Act was one the first twentieth-century civil rights laws designed to promote gender equity. Under the concept of comparable worth (tried relatively unsuccessfully on a limited scale in the United States and elsewhere in past decades), public entities attempted to equate dissimilar work done by men and women for pay equity purposes. For example, a female physical therapist might score the same number of comparable worth points as a male firefighter, mandating pay equity between their positions. Because such determinations inherently involve purely subjective value judgments, progress on the implementation of comparable worth was halted in recent decades, as it engenders more inequity than equity. Subsequent civil rights laws, such as Title VII of the Civil Rights Act of 1964 (prohibiting, among other forms of job discrimination, gender-based discrimination), serve this purpose better and more efficiently.[13]

The history of employee benefits, now an integral part of employee total compensation, is extremely interesting and illustrative of evolving values of equity and work-life balance. Before World War II, employee benefits largely did not exist. Few employees earned substantial vacation time or had individual or family health care insurance, retirement packages, continuing education support, or similar employment-related perks. After World War II, everything changed. What were formerly fringe benefits—that is, benefits that constituted only a few percentage points of total compensation—quickly evolved into benefit packages worth 20% to 40% of total compensation. In addition to the mandatory governmental benefits of Social Security, unemployment, and worker's compensation insurance, the benefits included such amenities as paid health and dental insurance, expansive vacation and global PTO (paid-time-off, including sick and personal days), child and elder care, and legal services. The ability to choose personalized permissive benefits packages resulted in the adoption of the term *cafeteria benefits.*

Why the growth in benefits packages for employees? In part, after World War II employees had greater opportunities for postsecondary education under the GI Bill. Also, employers and other members of society generally recognized the inherent value of employees as people and took on an important social responsibility role in this regard. The logical extension of that concept was the development of **employee assistance programs**, or EAPs. These confidential programs offer employees with substance abuse, psychological,[57,60] and marital or financial problems the opportunity to seek confidential assistance from third-party experts funded by the organization, before these problems inalterably damage the employees' careers.[36]

Incentives come in two categories: individual and work group incentives. An employee stock ownership plan is an example of a group incentive. An impact cash award given to a particular employee for merit is an example of an individual incentive. Incentives may be nonfinancial as well, such as certain impact awards that do not carry a monetary award with them. Incentives generally are designed to help employees develop an enhanced sense of self-worth and self-actualization and to improve worker productivity.

One form of incentive pay—variable (sliding-scale) compensation under managed care—gained notoriety over the past decade. Ethical issues involving the potentially divided loyalties of health care professionals who are paid large sums of money to save their managed care organizations substantial monetary outlays have led to governmental and consumer-group initiatives designed to curb abuse. At the very least, patients should be apprised, as part of the initial informed disclosure and consent process, that their primary health care providers may be receiving variable incentive pay incident to their care.

MANAGEMENT-LABOR RELATIONS

Management-labor relations is another core area within human resource managers' domain of jurisdiction. Human resource management specialists serve on management teams[9] in collective bargaining contract negotiations,[21,25,38] grievance processing, union representation elections, and related functions.

Not all management-labor relations involve what is commonly envisioned as conflict (e.g., union-management disputes). Management and **labor**, in unionized and nonunionized environments, cooperate closely much more often than they are in conflict.[31] For example, process action teams (PATs) are joint management-labor teams that tackle major and minor organizational problems. Peer review processes are similarly joint management-labor functions.

Unionization in physical therapy is an important issue. Although physical therapists have been legally empowered to unionize in all settings since 1974, they generally do not choose to do so. This election results in part from excellent relations with, and symbiosis between, professional labor and health management elements. The trend toward nonunionization is societal, too. From its twin heydays of the post-Depression–era 1930s and the carefree 1950s, when private sector unionization was at an all-time high of one third of the total workforce, it stood in 2006 at 12.5%, according to the Bureau of Labor Statistics.[10]

The cataclysmic event that led to the modern decline of private-sector unionization in the United States was the firing by President Reagan in 1981 of all federal air traffic controllers because of an illegal strike. The public simply did not, and does not now, sympathize with such actions by unions. For physical therapists, the dilemma of being represented by industrial unions and the ethical issues inherent in work stoppages contribute to the relative dearth of physical therapists who are unionized.

With the advent and rise of managed care, what has historically been close cooperation between health professionals and organizations is being strained to a certain degree. As a direct result of managed care, some disciplines—physicians, podiatrists, and nurses, in particular—have formed powerful, discipline focused unions to protect their members' interests. It remains to be seen whether physical therapy professionals follow suit.

Disciplinary and Grievance Procedures

Employee discipline is a critically important issue for physical therapy clinical managers and supervisors, one that they may feel unprepared to address. For reasons of patient and staff safety and orderly operations, however, management must maintain effective discipline.[30]

Discipline as a concept is broader in scope than counseling, which may involve formal or informal communication between managers and employees on the broadest range of topics, from enacting disciplinary measures to rewarding positive performance. Discipline involves the process of sanctioning employees for impermissible work-related behavior.

There are two general approaches to employee discipline: rehabilitative and punitive approaches. A rehabilitative, or constructive, approach to employee discipline focuses on undertaking remedial steps to encourage and effect desired work-related behaviors in employees. A punitive approach to employee discipline involves merely imposing punishment for undesirable employee behavior. From a human relations perspective (in place in most physical therapy clinical settings), a constructive approach to employee discipline is strongly recommended.

Under either approach to employee discipline, disciplinary action should be both progressive in nature and proportional to the offenses alleged. **Progressive discipline** entails utilizing a continuum of possible disciplinary measures to encourage compliance with official norms. At the outset, it is important that behavioral norms required of employees in clinical settings be clearly communicated to all employees so that they understand what is expected of them.

Depending on the offense, the continuum of employee discipline may include the following progressive measures:

1. Oral warning, under which an employee is apprised of the conduct warranting discipline and directed by management to conform to expected norms
2. Oral reprimand, a more formal process than the oral warning, under which an employee is given clear notice of the need to remediate his or her conduct
3. Written warning, a slightly more formal process than the oral reprimand, under which an employee is given notice of an infraction and the need to remediate behavior in writing
4. Written reprimand, under which more permanent documentation of the basis for employee discipline takes place
5. Withholding pay and/or benefits
6. Disciplinary suspension from the work setting, with or without pay
7. Disciplinary transfer and/or demotion in status
8. Discharge from employment, with or without severance pay or continuation of benefits other than those that are legally required
9. Turning over the evidence of criminal wrongdoing to law enforcement or licensing board officials[18,19]

In all cases of employee discipline, discipline should be carried out in private to safeguard the privacy rights of the disciplined employee and others who may be involved in the process (including patients, witnesses, and those who report possible infractions). Discipline inherently involves counseling, and a record of disciplinary counseling must be created and securely maintained. A disciplined employee should be asked to sign a record of counseling, and if he or she refuses, that refusal should be annotated on the counseling form. A sample counseling form appears in Figure 2-5.

For employees undergoing disciplinary counseling in a unionized environment, a **union representative** may have the right to be present, with or without the other parties' consent, pursuant to what is known in labor law as the **Weingarten rule**. This rule exists so that union interests are protected during employee disciplinary counseling. Human resource and clinical managers should consult with their facility attorneys for specific advice.

Scenarios that may lead to disciplinary action[6] against employees have recently been augmented by newly publicized ones, including résumé fraud and, according to Hicks, office romances. Hicks cited a 1993 Society for Human Resource Management survey showing that 90% of the Society's 65,000 human resource managers believe that office dating should not be prohibited, absent an existing superior-subordinate relationship between the parties.[29] Regarding résumé fraud, despite widespread written policies making this offense a basis for **dismissal**, dismissal is not normally carried out in practice, absent serious fraud.

The Society for Human Resource Management has called employment discharge a key issue for management. It and Korotkin recommended the procedural steps found in Box 2-7 when discharging employees.

ABC Health System

Anytown, USA

Employee Counseling Form

Note: This form is confidential. It may be reviewed only by the counselor, counseled employee, and supervisors in the counseled employee's direct chain of command, on a need-to-know basis. It is to be maintained in the employee's secure human resource file for a period not to exceed 3 years.

Date, time, and location of counseling:

Counselor:

Counseled employee:

Nature of counseling:

Employee input (if written, append to form):

Resolution/follow-up:

Signatures:

_____   _____
Counselor   Counseled employee

FIGURE 2-5 | Sample employee counseling form.

BOX **2-7** ▪ **Recommended Steps For Discharging Employees**[35,39]

1. Avoid on-the-spot discharges.
2. Conduct appropriate investigations of alleged offenses before taking final action, affording all key parties to an action the opportunity to be heard.
3. Consult proactively and on an ongoing basis with human resource and legal professionals for advice on how to proceed.
4. If discharge is deemed appropriate, notify the employee in person and cite a specific justifiable ground for the dismissal.
5. Retain documentation related to the discharge for the period of the statute of limitations for wrongful termination.

Employers are urged not to follow recent corporate examples of dismissal of employees via email notification.[55] This practice—purportedly carried out as part of a system-wide reduction in force—has been criticized by human resource management experts as dehumanizing to employees. The better approach to employee discharges incident to corporate downsizing is through face-to-face encounters with supervisors.

Another growing concern and basis for employee discipline is absenteeism, which is critically important for physical therapy because patient care can be directly and severely adversely affected by it. Vanderwall asserted that there has been a 25% increase in employee absenteeism across the board.[67] The most frequent reason cited is the quality-of-life issue of family obligations.

Regarding employees who voluntarily leave employment, Barada recommended that exit interviews be conducted to assess, in part, how to prevent similar losses of key employees in the future.[5] Such interviews should not be carried out on the day of discharge but rather 7 to 10 days thereafter, by a disinterested third party. The interviewer should project sincerity and empathy for the interviewee.

Managing a Diverse Workforce

It is without question that we live in a diverse world—at work, at play, at home, and elsewhere. Managers must be sensitive to cultural diversity in the workplace. Fully 88% of workforce growth over the next few decades will come from other than white males, according to Mathis.[44] Many states have in place laws requiring that English be spoken in the workplace. This law may violate civil rights legal protections of workers, absent any business necessity for requiring English in the workplace. Some 30 million Americans claim Spanish as their first language.

Everyone in physical therapy work settings and work settings in general must become culturally competent and embrace multiculturalism. Culture consists of norms, mores (values and formal practices), customs, and folkways, which are as disparate as are cultural groups and subgroups (including the culture within business organizations). Truly, the greatest attribute of the United States is its perceived, if not actual, tolerance of cultural diversity. From domestic partner benefits to affirmative action to religious accommodation, human resource managers are available for consultation and should be made an integral part of continuing education and professional development in this area.

SUMMARY

Unlike personnel management, which primarily addresses the inanimate inputs of production, human resource management addresses the individual and collective needs of people resources within an organization. Since the end of World War II, human resource management has been a recognized profession, with its own professional association and code of professional ethics. The seven classic human resource management functions include staffing; performance and competency assessment; compensation management; training and development; labor relations; safety, wellness and health programs management; and research. Physical therapy clinical managers should consult proactively with human resource management professionals to create and implement policies affecting staff within their organizations. Management by objectives, developed by Peter Drucker in 1954, is a philosophy under which a rated employee and his or her supervisor jointly develop, administer, and evaluate employee performance. Systematic employee training and development initiatives are key to optimal employee performance. Total compensation includes salaries or wages, benefits, and group and individual incentives. Optimization of management labor relations is critical for organizational success, whether in a unionized or nonunionized environment. Employee discipline may be either rehabilitative or punitive and should occur, when required, along a continuum of progressive measures, in a manner proportional to an offense.

REFERENCES AND READINGS

1. The Age Discrimination in Employment Act of 1967, 29 United States Code. Sections 621-634.
2. Amabile TM: How to kill creativity, *Harvard Business Review* 76(5): 76-87, 1998.
3. The Americans with Disabilities Act of 1990, Pub. L. No. 101-336 (1990) found at 42 USC. §§12101 et seq.
4. Apgar MIV: The alternative workplace: changing where and how people work, *Harvard Business Review* 76(3): 121-136, 1998.
5. Barada PW: Before you go, *HR Magazine* 43(12): 99-102, 1998.
6. Berglas S: Chronic time abuse, *Harvard Business Review* 82(6):90-97, 137, 2004.
7. Bernhard B: Shaping up: some employers now offering incentives to stay healthy, *San Antonio Express News* Jan. 22, 2006, 6N.
8. Bosman J: Stuck at the edges of the ad game: women feel sidelined in subtle ways, *New York Times* Nov. 22, 2005, C1, 5.
9. Brounstein M: *Managing teams for dummies,* Indianapolis, 2000, John Wiley and Sons.

10. Bureau of Labor Statistics: www.bls.gov. (Accessed Feb. 18, 2007.)
11. Challenger JE: Let prospective employer set interview agenda, *San Antonio Express News* Feb. 19, 2006, 2N.
12. Cherrington DJ: *The management of human resources,* ed 4, Englewood Cliffs, NJ, 1995, Prentiss-Hall, Inc.
13. Civil Rights Act of 1964, Title VII, 42 United States Code Section 703(e).
14. Clifton DW: *Physical rehabilitation's role in disability management: unique perspectives for success,* Philadelphia, 2004, Elsevier.
15. Conger JA: The necessary art of persuasion, *Harvard Business Review* 76(3): 84-95, 1998.
16. Coping with work-related stress, *San Antonio Express News* Apr. 23, 2006, 8S.
17. Digh P: *Religion in the workplace: make a good-faith effort to accommodate,* *HR Magazine* 43(12): 85-91, 1998.
18. Easterbals J: Drugs in the workplace, *HR Magazine* 43(2): 80-87, 1998.
19. Easterbals J: Dealing with drugs: keep it legal, *HR Magazine* 43(4): 104-116, 1998.
20. Equal Pay Act of 1963 (Pub. L. 88-38), Volume 29, United States Code Section 206(d).
21. Ertel D: Getting past yes: negotiating as if implementation mattered, *Harvard Business Review* 82(11): 60-68, 2004.
22. Falcone P: Rejuvenate your performance evaluation writing skills, *HR Magazine* 43(4): 104-116, 1998.
23. Fandray D: Getting things done, *Continental Magazine,* pp. 86-88, Oct. 2005.
24. Farmer J: Hiring staff in private practice, *PT Magazine* 12(9):46-49, Sept. 2004.
25. Fisher R, Ury W, Patton B: *Getting To yes,* London, 2001, Penguin.
26. Fleck C: Make the most of your experience, *AARP Bulletin,* pp. 18-19, Jan. 2006.
27. Goodman CK: Reverse mentoring now a workplace fact, *San Antonio Express News* May 7, 2006, 2G.
28. Grensing-Pophal L: Motivate managers to review performance, *HR Magazine,* pp. 44-48, Mar. 2001.
29. Hicks M: Love amid the cubicles, *San Francisco Examiner* Feb. 12, 1995, D1, D6.
30. Jeffrey C. The watched: who's zooming in on whom? *Mother Jones* 30(6): 26-27, 2005.
31. Kallick R: The résumé: an effective document increases job possibilities, *Health Careers Today,* pp. 6, 15, Feb. 2005.
32. Kinsman M: Workplace success often tied to social intelligence, *San Antonio Express News* May 21, 2006, 10R, 14N.
33. Kinsman M: The job interview dreaded by many, *San Antonio Express News* Apr. 23, 2006, 10R, 12R.
34. Kolb D, Williams J: Breakthrough bargaining, *Harvard Business Review* 78(2):89-97, Feb. 2000.
35. Korotkin MI: Damages in wrongful termination cases, *American Bar Association Journal,* pp. 84-87, May 1989.
36. Kriemer S: Psychologists find new role in the workplace, *San Antonio Express News* May 14, 2006, G2.
37. Krueger AB: Job satisfaction is not just a matter of dollars, *New York Times* Dec. 8, 2005, C3.
38. Lax DA, Sebenius JK: 3-D negotiation: playing the whole game, *Harvard Business Review,* 83(11):65-72, Nov. 2003.
39. Legal Report from the Society of Human Resource Management: Cardinal rules for disciplinary terminations, Alexandria, Va, 1995, Society for Human Resource Management.
40. Lencioni P: *Death by meeting,* San Francisco, 2004, Jossey-Bass.
41. Lewis K: Physical therapy contracts, *Clinical Management* 12(6):14-18, 1992.
42. Lohr S: How the game is played, *New York Times* Dec. 5, 2005, C1, 8.

43. Lubin JS: Some dos and don'ts to help you hone your videoconferencing skills, *Wall Street Journal* Feb. 7, 2006, B1.
44. Mathis RL, Jackson JH: *Human resource management,* ed 11, Cincinnati, 2005, Southwestern College Publishing.
45. Maruca RF: How do you manage an off-site team? *Harvard Business Review* 76(4): 22-35, 1998.
46. Mausy A: Web conferencing: smart tools for virtual meetings, *Texas Bar Journal* 66(11): 864, Nov. 2003.
47. McAtee DR III: Staying on top of your game, *Texas Bar Journal* 69(2):142-143, Feb. 2006.
48. McIntyre MG: New boss means new expectations, *San Antonio Express News* Apr. 16, 2006, G1.
49. Needleman SE: Be prepared when opportunity knocks, *Wall Street Journal* Feb. 7, 2006, B3.
50. Nero ME: Temp agencies becoming permanent solution, *San Antonio Express News* Jan. 22, 2006, 4N.
51. Orr C: Keys to success: how to make your resume digitally friendly, *San Antonio Express News: Keys to Success* Mar. 5, 2006, 3P.
52. Orr C: Women executives offer advice for success, *San Antonio Express News* Feb. 19, 2006, 6N.
53. O'Shea D: How to get your foot in the door for interview, *San Antonio Express News* Sept. 11, 2005, 3P.
54. Pavlik J: Working the office political machine, *Indianapolis Star* Sept. 12, 2004, F7.
55. Radio shack layoff notices are sent by e-mail, *New York Times* Aug. 31, 2006, C2.
56. Resume revival: simple ideas can pump new life into your job search, *San Antonio Express News* Jan. 22, 2006, 2N.
57. Romanski E: Physicians beat burnout: get a grip on stress before getting run down, *Humana's YourPractice,* p. 15, Fall 2004.
58. Rooke D, Torbert WR: 7 Transformations of leadership, *Harvard Business Review* 83(4): 66-76, 2005.
59. Sakis JR, Kennedy DB: Violence at work, *Trial,* 38(13): 32-36, Dec. 2002.
60. Scott RW: Manage stress so it doesn't manage you, *Risk Advisor,* p. 1, Summer 2000.
61. Scott RW: *Professional ethics: a guide for rehabilitation professionals,* St. Louis, 1998, Mosby.
62. Scott RW: *Promoting legal awareness in physical and occupational therapy,* St. Louis, 1997, Mosby.
63. Talk show: preparation key to success in interview, *San Antonio Express News* Mar. 19, 2006, 4P.
64. Tapping hidden networks improves chances of landing job, *San Antonio Express News* Apr. 23, 2006, 7R.
65. Thiruvengadam M: Sex, style and psychology, *San Antonio Express News* Jan. 1, 2006, 1L.
66. Turley WH: Psychological contract violations during corporate restructuring, *Human Resource Management* 37(2): 117-129, 1998.
67. Vanderwall S: Survey finds unscheduled absenteeism hitting seven-year high, *HR News,* p. 14, Nov. 1998.
68. Vedantam S: Home-work paradox persists, *Bangor Daily News* Sept. 4, 2006, A2.
69. Wallen E: A restrictive covenant can lessen a practice's risk of losing patients, *Physician's Financial News,* p. 26, May 1991.
70. Wells SJ: A new road: traveling beyond 360-degree evaluation, *HR Magazine* 44(9): 83-91, 1999.
71. Working for a competitor likely in today's economy, *San Antonio Express News* Apr. 9, 2006, 3M.

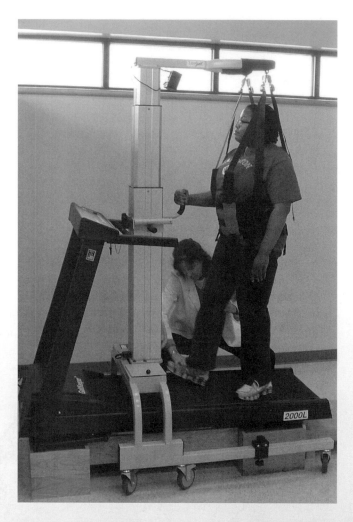

From Cameron MH, Monroe LG: *Physical rehabilitation*, St Louis, 2007, Saunders.

3

Physical Therapy Reimbursement and Financial Management

Christopher Petrosino

ABSTRACT

First and foremost, physical therapy is a hands-on health care profession that serves patients. However, without sustainable sources of revenue and financial stability maintained through prudent decision making, a physical therapy practice is at risk of closing. This chapter is designed to give managers a basic understanding of financial management in keeping with the opportunities and constraints of the health care milieu. An emphasis on financial management within the physical therapist continuum of care (PTCC) is the basis for addressing principles of reimbursement, accounting, budgeting, marketing, and business performance evaluation. The chapter begins by describing the history of health insurance and its relationship with physical therapy. The PTCC is emphasized as the basis for understanding site-specific reimbursement structures. The latter portion of the chapter is devoted to the basics of financial management for the physical therapist manager.

KEY WORDS AND PHRASES

Advanced beneficiary notice	Customary charges	Horizontal analysis
Appeal	Deductible	Income statement
Assets	Denials	Individualized education
Balance sheet	Diagnostic-related groups	program
Break-even analysis	Dividends	Liabilities
Budget	Durable medical equipment	Managed health care
Capital stock	Expense	Managerial accounting
Claims	Explanation of benefits	Market-based pricing
Coinsurance	Fiduciary	Minimum data set
Common-size statement	Financial management	Net income
Coordination of benefits	Financial statements	Net loss
Co-payment	Fixed cost	Owner's equity
Cost	Homebound	Prevailing charge
Cost-plus pricing	Home health resource	Price setting
Cost-volume-profit analysis	group	Primary care providers

Primary prevention
Profitability measures
Prospective payment
 system
Reasonable charge
Resource utilization
 groups
Retained earnings

Retained earnings
 statement
Retrospective payment
 system
Revenues
Secondary care providers
Secondary prevention
Semivariable cost

Solvency measures
Statement of cash flows
Tertiary care providers
Tertiary prevention
Third-party payment
 system
Variable cost
Vertical analysis

OBJECTIVES

1. Develop an understanding of reimbursement within the continuum of care and prevention.

2. Demonstrate knowledge of the history of health insurance as it relates to the development of the physical therapy profession.

3. Discern the relative advantages and disadvantages of the two primary health care payment systems.

4. Identify site-specific reimbursement systems in which physical therapists seek remuneration for services.

5. Be able to discuss the impact of managed care on physical therapy practice.

6. Identify the principal uses and users of financial information in the health care organization.

7. Practice ethically and legally when setting health care charge rates and when seeking third-party payer reimbursement.

8. Develop prudent and adequate departmental budgets to sustain operations and growth.

9. Assess key health care financial statements, suggesting areas of relative strength and weakness.

10. Evaluate the organization's financial health through the use of appropriate financial ratios.

11. Identify resources needed to gain a portion of the market share.

12. Apply the management principle of social responsibility to health care financial administration at the departmental, organizational, and systems levels.

HEALTH INSURANCE AND THE PHYSICAL THERAPY PROFESSION

During the second industrial revolution of the late 1800s, a few employers began offering employment-based health benefits to entice workers. As a result, the use of health care services increased. A trend in employment-based benefit, also known as *health insurance*, did not become prevalent until the National War Labor Board froze employee wages during World War I. World War I and the wage freeze caused a worker shortage and a need for employers to seek new ways to entice potential employees. During the early 1900s, group insurance plans began to emerge, and in 1912 the National Convention of Insurance Commissioners developed the first state law model to regulate health insurance. Employer payment of health insurance instituted what is now known as the **third-party payment system**.

In a third-party payment system, the patient or client is considered the first party or beneficiary, the second party is the one who provides the service (also known as the *provider*), and the third party is the private or governmental health insurance provider. This system has evolved to include companies contracting with a health insurance provider to pay the health care **claims** of their employees. A claim is the demand for something due or believed to be due.[1] Claims set the stage for **denials** from third-party payers, which are refusals to pay for services rendered. Typically, claims are disallowed when the third-party payer determines that the amount of a health care provider's charge exceeds a health insurance plan's coverage. A health care provider may request a review of the denial in which the accuracy of a third-party reimbursement is questioned. An **appeal** usually necessitates submitting additional information in support of the requested reimbursement. Clear coverage and limitations to insurance plans are established through a contractual agreement between the beneficiary and the payer. After each claim, the third-party payer submits an **explanation of benefits** (EOB) to the beneficiary and the provider in which coverage issues are addressed.

During the growth of the health insurance industry, the physical therapy profession was in its infancy as the United States Division of Special Hospitals and Physical Reconstruction began employing reconstruction aides in Army hospitals. The title *reconstruction aides*, used during wartime, was replaced by *physical therapists* as the profession became more established in hospitals during the 1920s. As health insurance programs began to take root, a **retrospective payment system** was established in which the provider is paid virtually all of its charges for services rendered. In this system, there is less incentive to control the **cost** of health care on the part of the providers, resulting in more services being provided to patients to procure greater **revenues** and profit. Because of the rising cost of health care, prepayment systems emerged. The first sustainable prepayment system was developed in 1929 at Baylor Hospital in Dallas, Texas. This prepayment system became a forerunner to the Blue Cross plans established in 1937.

Physical therapists weathered the financial hardships of the Great Depression through financial support from the Social Security Act of 1935, which provided governmental support for health care benefits, and the National Foundation for Infantile Paralysis (NFIP), which provided direct financial support to the profession.[2] Through World War II and the polio epidemic, the profession of physical therapy grew and hospital rehabilitation departments were considered financial profit centers. However, with the discovery of the Salk vaccine in 1955, which led to a dramatic decrease in the number of patients with polio, physical therapists began to worry about the life of the profession. Charles Magistro, PT, FAPTA, former president of the American Physical Therapy Association (APTA), estimated that 80% of physical therapy services were provided to patients with polio.[2] With the eradication of the disease and the withdrawal of financial support from the NFIP in 1962, the profession of physical therapy was obviously struggling. However, health care needs of the elderly and people with disability once again resulted in a financial boost to the physical therapy profession, in the form of governmental health insurance. Title XVIII and Title XIX of the Social Security Act were passed in 1965, establishing Medicare and Medicaid. The boon in health benefits and health care legislation continued with companies becoming self-insured (Firestone Tire and Rubber Co. 1968), the development of Health Maintenance Organizations (HMO Act of 1973), and the regulation of pension and welfare plans (Employee Retirement Income Security Act of 1974), which included health care benefits.

Unfortunately, health care costs skyrocketed in the retrospective payment system, putting a strain on the governmental health insurance system. The first sign of legislation to control costs occurred with the Deficit Reduction Act of 1984 (DEFRA), which made Medicare the secondary payer for covered health expenses of eligible enrollees between the ages of 65 and 69 who are covered by another health insurance plan. Rules for when more than one insurance plan covers a patient became established and were termed **coordination of benefits** (COB). Because a patient can have more than one insurance policy, the primary payer must make a judgment and settlement on a claim before a secondary insurer is required to consider payment. Typically, the governmental insurance plan would be the last insurance entity to incur the expense of the beneficiary's health care cost. Employee and dependent health care benefits were protected with the Consolidated Omnibus Budget Reconciliation Act of 1985 (COBRA), which allowed for continued benefits after termination of employment, and the Health Insurance Portability and Accountability Act of 1996 (HIPAA), which ensured nondiscrimination and the transferability of health care benefits after a change of employment.

The greatest impact on the physical therapy profession resulting from the government's attempt to control health care costs came in 1997 with the Balanced Budget Act (BBA). Although it created beneficial programs for children's health insurance, Medicare supplemental policies, and state regulation of Medicaid, the BBA had a devastating effect on physical therapy reimbursement and practice, with approximately 115 billion dollars cut from the Medicare program.[2] The Medicare Balanced Budget Refinement Act of 1999 rectified a portion of the health care reimbursement hardship by restoring an estimated 8 to 12 billion dollars to the Medicare program.[2] The BBA legislation set the stage for the government to control costs by initiating the replacement of the retrospective payment system with a **prospective payment system** (PPS).

A PPS is a method of reimbursement that determines payment to providers on the basis of a predetermined fixed amount. The payment amount is determined by a classification system that is specific to the health care setting and can be based on reimbursement per service, per visit, per case (or episode), or per enrollee. Through a PPS, the provider controls costs through the frugal use of resources. If the services are provided for less cost to the provider than the predetermined amount of reimbursement, the provider makes a greater profit, whereas when more resources are used to provide care and the cost of the service exceeds the predetermined amount, the provider loses money. Thus a provider is less likely to offer services that may be unnecessary to the patient's care. Sometimes, the incentive to minimize services and increase reimbursement results in inadequate care. Through the implementation of PPS to manage costs, quality, and access to health care, the federal government has demonstrated an effort to decrease the financial burden of governmental health insurance (Medicare and Medicaid) on taxpayers. With the need for the government to control health care spending through federal legislation and the implementation of PPS, **managed health care**, which had grown throughout the 1970s and 1980s, was brought to maturity in the 1990s.

Managed health care, implemented through managed care organizations (MCOs), is an attempt to control the cost of health care through provider networks; limitations on benefits to enrollees, including charging additional fees to enrollees for using out-of-network providers; and various systems of authorization for services. Managed care has evolved into a plethora of variations on third-party payment systems, from managed indemnity to preferred provider organizations (PPOs), point of service organizations, open-panel health maintenance organizations, and closed-panel health maintenance organizations. Regardless of the varying structures, the purpose of MCOs is to control the skyrocketing costs of health care. Health care professionals may argue that moving the financial risks from payers to providers through MCOs can hinder adequate and timely health care, create ethical concerns about appropriate care, encourage corporate profiteering, and endanger patients with exceptional needs who incur higher health care costs. In reality, there will always be a need to minimize the risk of unscrupulous acts, and all parties, including payers, providers, employers, and patients, have an implicit incentive to gain the best health care at the least cost, no matter which party has the most control over the financial gain or loss.

In an attempt to optimize financial gain and minimize financial loss, the physical therapist must be aware of the insurance coverage of each patient under his or her care. Likewise, regardless of setting, the physical therapist must appropriately document the services provided to justify payment. The APTA Code of Ethics[4] addresses reimbursement of physical therapy services in Principle 7: "A physical therapist shall seek only such remuneration as is deserved and reasonable for physical therapy services." The physical therapist or a designated staff member should contact the patient's insurance company whenever a question arises as to whether a service is covered and should follow up on denied claims in which a needed service was provided. The physical therapist will need to become recognized by the insurance company as a qualified provider to receive payment. Furthermore, patients must be made aware of their obligation to pay for any services that are not covered by the health insurance company. It is important for the physical therapist to realize that some patients may have poor health care coverage as a result of their financial situation whereas others may have poor coverage because they chose to assume a greater risk when selecting a health plan. Patients should carefully review each health insurance plan being offered by an employer or private insurance company and make a decision according to their assumed risk of illness or injury and their financial circumstances.

Patients, or beneficiaries, enter into a contractual agreement with the health insurance company, thereby agreeing to make payments in accordance with their policy when a covered event occurs or a covered service is provided by the physical therapist. It is important to note that the physical therapist should not negotiate fees with patients who have a contractual agreement with a third-party payer. By entering into an agreement with a third-party payer, the patient has agreed to assume a level of risk and will need to pay in accordance with the policy and any charges that are not covered. Typically, an enrollee will pay a yearly premium for a health care insurance policy. In corporate health plans, the premium is most often

automatically deducted from the employee's salary. The policy may include a
deductible, which is an amount of money that is required to be paid out of pocket
by the enrollee before the insurance begins to cover any medical expenses. The
deductible is typically reinstated each year. Most health insurance policies also have
co-payments or **coinsurance** that the patient has agreed to pay out of pocket.
A co-payment is a fixed amount of money paid directly to the service provider by the
enrollee that is typically collected upon arrival at each visit. Coinsurance is a provision
in a health insurance policy that limits the amount of coverage in a plan by a certain
percentage (e.g., 80%) and in which the remaining percentage is paid out of pocket
by the enrollee (e.g., 20%). Upon admission or arrival for an initial physical therapy
evaluation, a staff member should review the patient's medical insurance card and
clarify coverage. The patient, provider, and third-party payer should have an
understanding of the enrollee's coverage and resolve any conflicting information as
soon as a concern is identified. Government health insurance, Medicare B, has even
instituted a rule called an **advanced beneficiary notice** (ABN), which obligates the
provider to inform the patient when Medicare will not cover a service and the patient
can be directly billed. Regardless of health care setting, a physical therapist must
understand each patient's health insurance coverage to best serve the patient, make
appropriate clinical decisions based on insurance parameters, and document within
the required guidelines to receive reimbursement for services provided.

The physical therapy manager has the additional responsibility of ensuring that
each therapist is aware of documentation and billing requirements in order to
provide quality care and seek deserved remuneration. With health care
reimbursement in constant flux, the physical therapist manager must also be
attentive and responsive to changes in third-party payer reimbursement, legislation
at state and federal levels affecting reimbursement, and site-specific changes in the
company's billing or reimbursement policies and procedures. The successful growth
of the physical therapy profession depends in part on the ability of the physical
therapist to influence reimbursement policies and adapt to change within the
dynamic health care reimbursement milieu.

EXERCISE 3-1

Read your own health insurance policy. Bring the policy to class, and, in pairs, compare
coverage in regard to what is covered and what is not. Compare deductibles, co-payments,
and coinsurance. How does the policy address pre-existing conditions, access to
specialists, preventive care services, and pre-authorization? What coverage is offered for
physical therapy services? How do the exclusions and limitations of the policy affect physical
therapy services? If you are in an MCO, what is their policy on going "out of network"?

CONTINUUM OF CARE

Health care reimbursement often defines the extent of care that a patient can receive
from a health care provider. Without reimbursement, care of the patient is quickly

reduced to meeting basic needs, providing instruction in care to the patient or caregiver, and discharging the patient from the health care setting. Likewise, the setting in which a patient receives physical therapy care can be determined by a patient's classification of disablement and the available reimbursement to the provider of care. Frequently, a physical therapist must make an ethical decision about the level of care for a patient by considering appropriate health care setting, available reimbursement, caregiver support, living situation, and a variety of other factors. Through the collection and synthesis of information about the patient's life situations, the physical therapist decides where the patient would best be served.[6] Services provided by health care professionals are considered to be on a continuum depending on the patient's point of entry into the health care system and discharge destinations for further care, as well as the roles assumed by the health care practitioners.

The continuum of care is often invoked by care providers but seldom operationally defined for meaningful use in a health care discipline. The *Guide to Physical Therapist Practice*[2] provides a good starting point for understanding the continuum of care for physical therapist practice by defining the role of the physical therapist in primary, secondary, and tertiary care and prevention. Considering the utility of classifying the level of care required to meet specific patient needs, Petrosino (CLP, unpublished data, 2006) developed the Physical Therapy Continuum of Care (PTCC) model (Figure 3-1). The PTCC model defines six intervention levels of physical therapist patient care with regard to contact time with patients, patient dependence, the role of the physical therapist, and the health care setting.

The classification system is intended to assist in clinical decision making about the appropriate level of physical therapist intervention and the appropriate care facility to provide those services. Through use of terminology from the *Guide to Physical Therapist Practice* and the *International Classification of Functioning, Disability, and Health (ICIDH-2)*, the PTCC integrates the physical therapist's role in primary, secondary, and tertiary care and prevention to develop a coding system within the levels of intervention and across a practice setting continuum. Each level of intervention is defined in consideration of contemporary practice and is considered a dynamic model in need of updates reflecting all significant changes in the provision of health care. Based on the patient's/client's impairment, functional limitations, disability, and financial resources, the model is intended to provide an approach to understanding the role of a physical therapist in the continuum of care, as well as a framework to assist in selecting an appropriate practice setting for a patient or client.

There are six levels of intervention in the PTCC model. Each level of intervention calls into consideration the progression of the patient/client from dependence to independence in overcoming impairments, functional limitations, and disability. Although the progression from inpatient to outpatient to patient in a community-based practice setting is plausible, it is not obligatory; the patient/client can enter the continuum at any level and move up or down levels depending on improvement in function or a decline in his or her ability to perform. Table 3-1 lists the individual settings within each of the six levels of the PTCC model.

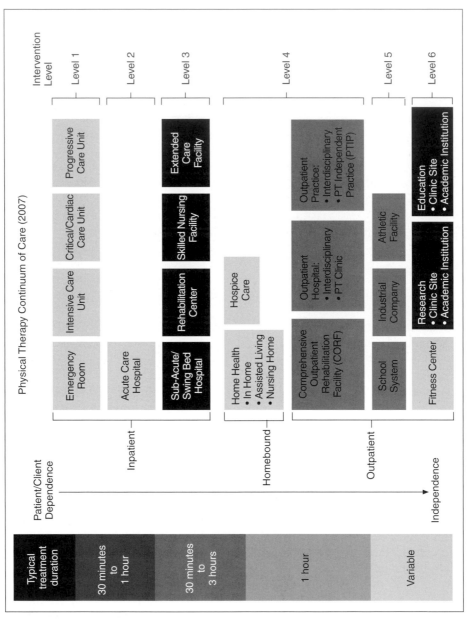

Physical Therapy Continuum of Care (2007)

Intervention Level

- Level 1
- Level 2
- Level 3
- Level 4
- Level 5
- Level 6

Progressive Care Unit

Critical/Cardiac Care Unit

Intensive Care Unit

Emergency Room

Acute Care Hospital

Sub-Acute/Swing Bed Hospital

Extended Care Facility

Skilled Nursing Facility

Rehabilitation Center

Hospice Care

Home Health
- In Home
- Assisted Living
- Nursing Home

Outpatient Practice:
- Interdisciplinary
- PT Independent Practice (PTIP)

Outpatient Hospital:
- Interdisciplinary
- PT Clinic

Comprehensive Outpatient Rehabilitation Facility (CORF)

Athletic Facility

Industrial Company

School System

Education
- Clinic Site
- Academic Institution

Research
- Clinic Site
- Academic Institution

Fitness Center

Patient/Client Dependence

Inpatient

Homebound

Outpatient

Independence

Typical treatment duration

30 minutes to 1 hour

30 minutes to 3 hours

1 hour

Variable

FIGURE 3-1 | Physical therapy continuum of care.

TABLE 3-1 INDIVIDUAL SETTINGS WITHIN EACH OF THE SIX LEVELS OF THE PTCC MODEL

PTCC Level	Setting
Level 1-1	Emergency Room
Level 1-2	Intensive Care Unit
Level 1-3	Critical/Cardiac Care Unit
Level 1-4	Progressive Care Unit
Level 2-1	Acute Care Facility
Level 3-1	Sub-Acute Unit or Swing Hospital
Level 3-2	Rehabilitation Center
Level 3-3	Skilled Nursing Facility
Level 3-4	Extended Care Facility
Level 4-1	Home Health Agency
Level 4-2	Hospice Care
Level 4-3	Comprehensive Outpatient Rehab Facility
Level 4-4	Outpatient Hospital
Level 4-5	Outpatient Practice
Level 5-1	School System
Level 5-2	Industrial Company
Level 5-3	Athletic Facility
Level 6-1	Fitness Center
Level 6-2	Research
Level 6-3	Education

When determining a patient's level on the PTCC, first consider his or her point of entry into the health care system (i.e., the setting in which the first physical therapy initial evaluation was performed) and the physical therapy intervention needed. Intervention Level 1 typically requires 30 to 60 minutes of direct contact treatment time by the physical therapist or physical therapist assistant at each physical therapy session. With consideration of the components of physical therapy intervention defined in the *Guide* (i.e., coordination, communication, and documentation; patient/client-related instruction; procedural interventions), Level 1 treatment interventions are focused on promoting patient safety, preventing loss of function, creating a healing environment, and optimizing potential for function. Currently, there are four settings classified under Level 1, and they are designated by the corresponding numbers 1 through 4.

Level 1

Level 1-1, the Emergency Room (ER), is equipped for the reception and treatment of persons requiring immediate medical care.[1] After receiving care in the ER, the patient may be released home, held for observation, or admitted to the acute care setting. In the past, ER care given by the physical therapist was limited to wound care and the disbursement and instruction in the use of **durable medical equipment** (DME; e.g., crutches, walkers, arm slings). Physical therapy services and consulting expertise are increasingly prevalent in the ER setting, with some hospitals assigning a physical therapist to the ER and billing for units of services provided. Level 1-2, the Intensive Care Unit (ICU), requires admission to the hospital and is used for continuous monitoring and treatment of seriously injured or ill patients using special medical equipment and services. Level 1-3, the Critical Care Unit or Cardiac Care Unit (CCU), is typically used for patients with specific diagnoses who are expected to have an abrupt change for the better or worse and who require close monitoring. Level 1-4, the Progressive Care Unit (PCU), is used as a step-down unit between intensive or critical care units and the acute care setting. Being admitted to an ICU, CCU, or PCU is considered an acute care stay, and patients can be categorized by **diagnostic-related groups** (DRG) for billing third-party payers, specifically Medicare. As part of the PPS for inpatient hospital care, DRGs are a way of classifying patients into payment categories according to diagnosis. Each patient episode of injury or illness will have a fixed fee regardless of the cost incurred by the hospital. Table 3-2 summarizes the reimbursement structure for each of the six levels of the PTCC model.

Level 2

PTCC Level 2-1, Acute Care (AC), is the only setting classified under Intervention Level 2 and has the number one as its designator. Intervention Level 2 typically requires 30 to 60 minutes of direct contact treatment time by the physical therapist or physical therapist assistant per physical therapy session, and treatments may be required twice a day (BID). Level 2-1 is characterized by interventions focused on minimizing functional limitations, educating patients for safety and function, and optimizing recovery after illness, injury, or surgery through working on functional mobility. For governmental health insurance (e.g., Medicare), DRGs are used in the AC setting to classify patients for case-based reimbursement.

Level 3

PTCC Level 3 is considered the most intensive, hands-on level of physical therapy services. Clients can require 30 minutes to 3 hours of direct contact treatment time by the physical therapist or physical therapist assistant each day. Physical therapy interventions at this level are focused on restoring or optimizing function for self-care, home management, return to work, return to community activities, or return to leisure activities. There are four settings identified under Level 3, and all Level 3 settings require an inpatient admission to the respective facility with specific criteria for patient admission. Level 3-1, Sub-acute Care or Swing Bed Hospital, is a step-down unit from AC in facilitating the client's transition to either return home or move to a more intensive rehabilitation facility. Level 3-2 is an Inpatient

TABLE 3-2 SUMMARY OF THE REIMBURSEMENT STRUCTURE FOR EACH OF THE SIX LEVELS OF THE PTCC MODEL

Level	Focus of Physical Therapy Intervention	Practice Setting	Government Reimbursement Classification System (Medicare)	Unit of Payment
1	Safety; healing environment; prevent loss of function; assist in stabilizing the patient condition	Emergency room	CPT codes; Physician Fee Schedule (PFS; based on Resource Based Relative Value System)	Per service
		Intensive care unit	Diagnostic-related groups	Per episode
		Critical care unit	Diagnostic-related groups	Per episode
		Progressive care unit	Diagnostic-related groups	Per episode
2	Minimize functional limitations; improve mobility; provide education for safety; increase independence	Acute care	Diagnostic-related groups	Per episode
3	Restore function; minimize impairment; improve mobility; increase independence	Sub-acute care/swing bed hospital	MDS: Resource Utilization Groups	Per case
		Rehabilitation	IRF-PAI: Case Mix Groups	Per case
		Skilled nursing facility	MDS: Resource Utilization Groups	Per case
		Extended care facility	MDS: Resource Utilization Groups	Per case

Continued

TABLE 3-2 SUMMARY OF THE REIMBURSEMENT STRUCTURE FOR EACH OF THE SIX LEVELS OF THE PTCC MODEL—CONT'D

Level	Focus of Physical Therapy Intervention	Practice Setting	Government Reimbursement Classification System (Medicare)	Unit of Payment
4	Increase, maintain, or restore function; improve quality of life; improve activity tolerance; improve independence in basic activities of daily living	Home Health	OASIS: Home Health Resource Group	60 day episode of care
		Hospice	CPT codes; payment determined by the hospice pricer	Per service
		Comprehensive outpatient rehabilitation facility	CPT codes; Physician Fee Schedule	Per service
		Outpatient hospital	CPT codes; Physician Fee Schedule	Per service
		Outpatient practice	CPT codes; Physician Fee Schedule	Per service
5	Improve independence in instrumental, vocational, or avocational activities	School system	Individual educational plan; school district tax levy and supplement from the government (Medicaid)	Per case
		Industrial company	Varies in accordance with self-insured company or state worker's compensation	Per episode or per service
6	Assist others in optimizing health and functional abilities, preventing impairment, and promoting function	Athletic facility	Facility funded or private insurance	Covered by the facility or per service
		Fitness center	Fee for service out-of-pocket	Per service
		Research	Primarily retrospective payment Grant funded (internal or external; public or private)	Funded by facility or grant
		Education	Grant funded (internal or external; public or private)	Funded by clinic or academic institution

Rehabilitation Facility (IRF), in which a minimum of 3 hours of treatment per day is required per patient and the patient must meet criteria for admission. Considered the most intense physical therapy care setting, the PPS for IRFs requires that 75% of a facility's patient population meet one or more specified pathological conditions of admission. The patient's functional levels are documented on the Inpatient Rehabilitation Facility—Patient Assessment Instrument (IRF—PAI), which is used to classify patients into distinct groups based on clinical presentation and resource utilization.[5] Separate payments are calculated for each case mix group to determine reimbursement.

Level 3-3 are Skilled Nursing Facilities (SNFs), licensed institutions providing skilled nursing care. SNFs have equivalent Medicare reimbursement requirements as swing-bed hospitals, which require physical therapists to document treatment minutes on the **minimum data set** (MDS). The MDS is an assessment instrument used in SNFs to classify patients by case into **resource utilization groups** (RUGs). RUG categories for rehabilitation are based on minutes of treatment time and appropriate disciplines being involved in the patient care. Although classified as different settings in the PTCC because of different regulatory requirements, SNFs and Level 3-4, Extended Care Facilities (ECFs; nursing or convalescent homes that offers skilled nursing and rehabilitation services), have the same reimbursement requirements for Medicare.

Level 4

Patients at Level 4 have been discharged home, although not all of them are able to care for themselves or function adequately in the home or community. At Levels 4-1 and 4-2, patients are discharged home but are considered **homebound**. *Homebound* literally means "confined to the home" and does not constitute ambulatory care. Level 4-1 includes services provided by home health agencies (HHAs). The HHA PPS for Medicare is based on a 60-day episode of care and a case mix adjustment as determined by documentation on the Outcome and Assessment Information Set (OASIS). Information from OASIS is used to assign patients into a **home health resource group** (HHRG) that determines the payment rate the HHA will receive. The intent of intervention for home health care is to promote greater independent function in the home and help the patient progress to ambulatory care if possible. Level 4-2, Hospice Care, is palliative care to maintain comfort levels in patients who are terminally ill. Payment for Hospice Care is determined by the Hospice Cap and Hospice Wage Index, which is updated yearly. A computer software program called Hospice Pricer determines reimbursement per service. Direct contact treatment interventions by the physical therapist or physical therapist assistant for Levels 4-1 and 4-2 typically range from 30 minutes to 1 hour. Level 4-3 begins ambulatory care services in which physical therapy can be provided without a patient being admitted to a health care facility or required to be homebound. The Comprehensive Outpatient Rehabilitation Facility (CORF), Level 4-3, is a Medicare-certified facility that is reimbursed on a fee-for-service basis through private or governmental insurance. A CORF differs from other outpatient clinics in that it is required to provide multidisciplinary services with the minimal complement of services provided by a physical therapist, physician, social worker, and psychologist or psychiatrist. Outpatient hospitals, Level 4-4, or privately owned outpatient practices, Level 4-5, may have interdisciplinary services or provide the services of one discipline and are also reimbursed on a fee-for-service basis. Services within PTCC Level 4 typically require 1 hour of direct contact time with the physical therapist or physical therapist assistant per treatment intervention.

Level 5

Intervention Level 5 of the PTCC is reserved for specialized settings in which physical therapy services are required to improve performance or independence (or both) in instrumental, vocational, or avocational activities. As with most categories of Level 4, Level 5 treatment interventions typically require 1 hour of hands-on care by the physical therapist or the physical therapist assistant. Level 5-1 incorporates school systems into the PTCC model. Governed by the Individuals with Disabilities Education Improvement Act of 2004 (IDEIA), children who are eligible for governmental funding for physical therapy services in school systems must have an **individualized education program** (IEP). An IEP is a multidisciplinary plan to improve educational results of children with disabilities. The IEP is updated yearly and developed through the collaboration of parents, students, and professionals from multiple disciplines. Programs such as the IEP are typically supported through a school district tax levy, with some support coming from federal- and state-regulated health care programs (e.g., Medicaid). Level 5-2 addresses the industrial setting and workers' compensation programs. The intent of physical therapy intervention for workers is to return them to gainful employment, preferably to the position they held before the injury or illness. In most states, companies can buy workers' compensation insurance from private insurance companies, although some states (e.g., Ohio, West Virginia) offer only a state-run workers' compensation program. Each state workers' compensation program has its own rules regarding processing claims and seeking reimbursement. Reimbursement to providers is typically based on a PPS fee-for-service basis, and the provider can purchase an information manual from the state that delineates fee schedules and code lists. Level 5-3 takes into account athletic facilities, traditionally at the high-school, college, and professional levels. The physical therapist's role in the athletic setting is to return patients to their chosen sport or improve the athlete's performance. Private insurance on a fee-for-service basis is the most common type of reimbursement for athletes, but sponsors of the athlete, owners of the athletic team, affiliated companies, or the athlete may hire providers to perform rehabilitation, performance testing, or physical training.

Level 6

The final level on the PTCC is Level 6, which encompasses primarily preventive care, health promotion, wellness, and the promotion of evidence-based practice in physical therapy for the betterment of patients/clients. The direct contact time of physical therapy interventions at this level varies widely, as do the reimbursement structures. For Level 6-1, fitness centers, physical therapists are the providers of choice as experts in exercise. Physical therapists have the knowledge base and skills to improve patients'/clients' functional limitations caused by injury or illness, establish normal function, and optimize performance in a fitness center setting. Level 6-2, research sites, addresses the need for physical therapists to embrace research in the academic and clinical settings to provide support for the efficacy of examination and treatment procedures. Research assists with justification for the profession and third-party payment. Funding for research initiatives primarily comes from internal and external grants provided by private or governmental institutions or agencies. Level 6-3, education sites, addresses educational services provided for patients or the professional development of health care workers. Physical therapists often provide educational programs or inservices without a fee (i.e., pro bono) for altruistic or marketing purposes. Occasionally, an honorarium is given to the speaker in appreciation of a community presentation or lecture in a continuing education course. The speaker may also charge a fee for the service provided. Most insurance companies do not reimburse for wellness and prevention education, although some employers do reimburse employees for participating in continuing education courses. Academic faculty is another career track for physical therapists with appropriate experience and postprofessional academic degrees. Academic faculty members are typically open to providing information about current interventions to clients seeking advice.

After determining the level at which the patient/client enters the PTCC and reviewing the interventions and reimbursement structure at that level, the physical therapist's role in the care and prevention of known or potential impairments, functional limitations, disabilities, or changes in health status should be considered. As **primary care providers**, physical therapists work in health care teams and provide services throughout the patient's life span, from pediatrics to geriatrics, addressing health care needs that involve impairment, functional limitation, disabilities, and changes in health status. The doctoring profession of physical therapy has positioned physical therapists as high-quality health care providers within the profession's scope of practice who are competent in coordinating and integrating the provision of services by referral to other disciplines when the patient's needs are beyond the scope of physical therapy practice. As **secondary care providers**, physical therapists accept referrals from other health care providers when physical therapy interventions are warranted. Physical therapists accept referrals in all health care settings on the PTCC as well as in other contemporary practice settings. As **tertiary care providers**, physical therapists provide consultation and other specialized services for patients/clients, families, corporations, and other health care providers. One of the primary roles of the physical therapist is that of an educator. In the PTCC model, the role of the physical therapist in patient care is designated as *a* for primary care, *b* for secondary care, and *c* for tertiary care. The care designator follows the setting designation. For example, a physical therapist providing consultation services to nursing staff in an AC hospital regarding the appropriate gait pattern for a patient who is status post open reduction internal fixation (ORIF) of the left femur would be classified as PTCC Level 2-1c. The numeral *2* indicates the intervention level by the physical therapist on the PTCC, the *1* after the dash indicates the AC hospital setting, and the letter *c* indicates tertiary care provided by the therapist.

Physical therapists are also involved in primary, secondary, and tertiary prevention. **Primary prevention** addresses health promotion efforts and education provided by the physical therapist for relatively healthy individuals who may be susceptible to a specific condition. **Secondary prevention** is accomplished by early physical therapy diagnosis and intervention for patients/clients with an identified or unidentified medical condition that is susceptible to a longer duration of illness, a progression in severity of disease or injury, or further impairment or functional limitations without physical therapist intervention. **Tertiary prevention** is physical therapist interventions to limit the severity of disability and functional limitations in patients with chronic and irreversible injuries or illnesses. In the PTCC model, the designator *x* is used for primary prevention, *y* for secondary prevention, and *z* for tertiary prevention (Table 3-3). The prevention designator follows the care designator in the PTCC model to complete identification of extent of care provided by the physical therapist using the PTCC model. Continuing with the aforementioned example, the physical therapist would be involved in secondary prevention and the complete PTCC model designation would be PTCC Level 2-1cy.

The PTCC model is used primarily to assist in understanding the physical therapist's role in the continuum of care, provide a basic knowledge and starting point for further investigation of setting-specific reimbursement for physical therapy students, and act as a discussion catalyst for students pursuing a doctorate in physical therapy. Furthermore, the PTCC model could be useful in decision making when planning a patient discharge from one setting or intervention level to the next. Jette, Grover, and Keck determined that decision making in discharge placement after a stay in an AC setting takes into consideration the patient's functioning and disability, wants and needs, ability to participate, and biopsychosocial environment in addition to the therapist's experience, the sharing of opinions within the health care team, and health care regulations.[6,18] With specific considerations regarding the individual patient and subsequent influencing factors such as those identified by Jette, Grover, and Keck,[18] delving into the specifics of a certain PTCC level may clarify appropriate discharge options for the patient. The efficacy of the PTCC model as a teaching tool is currently under investigation.

TABLE 3-3 DESIGNATORS FOR LEVEL OF CARE AND PREVENTION

a = primary care	x = primary prevention
b = secondary care	y = secondary prevention
c = tertiary care	z = tertiary prevention

EXERCISE 3-2

A) With the information provided, attempt to classify the following scenario into a PTCC level:

A 7-year-old boy named Jason, who was diagnosed with cerebral palsy at 6 months of age, arrives at the physical therapy independent practice where you work. Jason was injured in a bicycle accident in which he sustained a fracture of his distal humerus. The cast on his right arm was removed 1 week ago, and Jason has impaired range of motion at the elbow with a functional limitation in his ability to dress himself, a limitation resulting from pain in his elbow.

B) Discuss with a partner the appropriate PTCC level of classification. Collaborate with your partner to modify the scenario and move one level up or down on the PTCC. In consideration of the change in PTCC level, change the role of the therapist in the type of care given, and then change the role of the therapist in the type of prevention given.

C) Select one of the partners to present your modified scenario to the class. Did any classmates develop similar scenarios?

D) Discuss the benefits and limitations of using the PTCC model.

FINANCIAL MANAGEMENT AND PRICING

Keeping up to date on health insurance policies and specific reimbursement changes is critical in ensuring prudent financial decision making and optimizing the potential for success of the physical therapy practice. A physical therapist manager must effectively use financial information to assess the practice's financial status and health, fiscal efficiency and efficacy of employees, and compliance with internal and organizational budgetary controls. The physical therapist manager must act as a **fiduciary** to the clinic and organization. A fiduciary is a person entrusted to act in the best interests of the organization. **Financial management** can be defined as the gathering and proper use of financial information to plan, develop, implement, direct, and evaluate the activities of a physical therapy practice. Physical therapy financial management is the primary responsibility of physical therapist clinical managers for their domains of operations. Financial management encompasses general fiscal planning and control; budgetary development, approval, and implementation; funding of operational and nonoperational endeavors; reimbursement management; and facilities planning and development. A first step in financial management of a physical therapy practice is gathering and understanding financial information.

Determining what fee to charge per service, also called **price setting**, is a reasonable starting point in understanding physical therapy finances. A charge for a service is typically called a *fee*, whereas a charge for goods, such as DME, is called a *price*. Physical therapists charge fees for provided services to gain reimbursement from third-party payers. The pricing method chosen can be based on capitation (i.e., setting a limit that the service fee will not exceed), bundling (i.e., fee rates set per visit or per case), per unit of time, or per treatment application.

In **market-based pricing**, the reimbursement for a service should be considered customary, prevailing, and reasonable. **Customary charges** are determined by a median charge that providers request for the specific service. **Prevailing charges** assess charges according to a high percentage (e.g., 90%) of what providers consider to be customary in a geographical area. A **reasonable charge** is the lowest charge that covers the cost of the service with a profit for providing the service. In using market-based pricing, caution must be taken not to set prices in collusion with other providers, a practice that results in restraint of trade and potential violation of antitrust laws. Another common way to develop a charge per service is to first consider the estimated cost of a service or product (inclusive of manpower, supplies, overhead, procurement, storage, disbursal, etc.) in addition to a reasonable percentage of that cost figure for gross earnings (e.g., net of taxes and other indirect expenses), plus a reasonable profit. This method of cost analysis is sometimes called **cost-plus pricing**. To use cost-plus pricing, the manager must determine how cost changes in relation to providing the service (i.e., cost behavior). Costs can be considered fixed, variable, or semivariable. **Fixed costs** do not change in relation to the volume of service provided. For example, a pediatric physical therapy practice that buys a developmental motor test for toddlers will incur a fixed cost for the test. Regardless of the number of developmental motor tests performed, the cost of the test is fixed. **Variable cost** may increase or decrease with the amount of the service provided. For example, the cost of supplies varies according to the amount used on patients who require wound care. In other words, if you have an increased volume of such patients, the cost for wound care supplies (e.g., 4 × 4s, dressings, sterile gloves, suture kits) not billed to the patient would increase, causing an increased cost for providing the service. **Semivariable costs** have both fixed and variable costs associated with providing the service. An example of a semivariable cost is when a physical therapy clinic purchases a functional capacity evaluation (FCE) package. The price for performing an FCE would need to include the fixed cost of buying the equipment and the variable cost of a service charge from the FCE provider for software use (e.g., reports, billing, database information) on a per evaluation basis. The cost-volume relationship can be used to assess when the volume of service provided equals the cost of the service and thereby determine the break-even point at which any further service would provide a profit. The **break-even analysis** determines the point of volume at which total revenue equals total cost. For instance, if the cost of a pediatric development test is $500 (fixed cost), the cost of administering the test by the therapist is $35 (variable cost), and the practice is charging $100 for the service, then we can calculate that approximately eight patients would need to receive the evaluation of the test for the practice to make a profit. The break-even point is derived from the following equation:

Break-Even Point = Total Fixed Cost/[Price-Variable Cost]

The previous example demonstrates a break-even point that could be relevant in deciding whether to purchase the pediatric developmental test in light of how much it will be used and when it will generate a profit. Nonetheless, providing the best patient care should weigh heavily in the purchase decision. On a larger scale, the total revenues from the services provided and equipment sold in the practice can be compared with the total costs (fixed costs + variable costs + semivariable costs) to determine the break-even point at which an operating profit for the business will be achieved. This analysis method, called a **cost-volume-profit analysis**, is typically represented graphically and provides information that can be used to set fees for services, determine types of services to offer, perform real or simulated comparative analysis of changes in costs on profit for decision making, or develop a marketing strategy.

There are other methods of establishing a price for a service that are beyond the scope of this text (e.g., demand-minus pricing, marginal cost pricing, mark-up pricing, target pricing) and different pricing strategies used to gain a share of the market. All pricing methods share the need for a clear description of the charge, a unit of measure (e.g., per procedure or per intervention time), a price, and a code used for billing. Furthermore, the understanding of cost behavior and break-even analysis provides a foundation for financial decision making and conducting a cost-volume-profit analysis.

In lieu of other price-setting methods, some physical therapy managers use the governmental PPS to assist in setting charges. The Medicare PPS for outpatient clinics is based on the Physician Fee Schedule (PFS), which classifies services into Common Procedural Terminology codes (CPT code) that have a monetary value assigned to the code. The American Medical Association (AMA) developed CPT codes for use by public and private providers and third-party payers to report services and seek reimbursement. Editorial and advisory panels of the AMA create, refine, and delete codes. Although the codes are not considered to be specific to particular health care disciplines (i.e., all recognized health care providers can use the codes for billing), the most common codes used by physical therapists are in the 97000 series of the physical medicine and rehabilitation section. The Centers for Medicare and Medicaid Services (CMS), which regulate the governmental health insurance program, adopted the Resource-Based Relative-Value System (RBRVS) to assign charges to CPT codes. The RBRVS allows payments to be determined by the costs and resources needed to provide the service classified by a CPT code. Each code is given a relative value that takes into consideration the provider's work value, the expense of running the practice (e.g., labor, facility expenses, supplies), and the cost of professional liability (malpractice) expenses. A conversion factor that is based on economic factors is also used in determining Medicare Part B payment. In accordance with the amount determined by the PFS, Medicare will not pay any charges for that service above the predetermined amount attached to the CPT code. Some procedures are subject to code edits that restrict the ability of the physical therapist to bill for certain procedures in the same session. Other services are bundled into a single code restricting the ability to bill for the services separately. Likewise, modifiers can be used to provide clarification and further information about the distinct procedural services that warrant reimbursement. Physical therapy managers are responsible for ensuring that each practitioner under their supervision is knowledgeable about the proper coding, edits, bundling, and modifiers to optimize reimbursement and reduce denial rates. Oversight of physical therapist billing is a fiduciary duty of the manager even when each individual therapist is certified as a Medicare provider, which assumes the therapist's responsibility in billing.

Once a charge is determined for each service, all charges are developed into a fee schedule for the practice. A fee schedule is a list of services provided by the physical therapist and their corresponding charges. Although it is easier to manage one fee schedule, multiple fee schedules are legal in most states. Multiple fee schedules are typically considered because of varying allowed fees from third-party payers, coverage limits, and attempts to accommodate patients who do not have the financial resources to purchase a sufficient health insurance plan. This practice creates a gap between the charge for physical therapy services and the amount reimbursed by various third-party payers. In light of this gap, most states have legalized multiple fee schedules. Even if multiple fee schedules are legal, the therapist should still review the limitations of the third-party payer contracts for any potential breach and have a system in place to consistently bill the reasonable and appropriate charge for the patient and payer. With multiple fee schedules, care must be taken not to violate the Robinson-Patman Act of 1936, which prohibits businesses from charging similar customers different prices unless the differences are based on real cost differences. Some physical therapists opt to manage the multiple fees by using one list of fees and providing discounts in accordance with various payer agreements. Other physical therapy managers opt to hire, or consult regularly with, a reimbursement specialist to ensure compliance with ever-changing federal and private payer rules while managing multiple fee schedules.

Because of allowable charges by third-party payers, the amount received by the provider is rarely the price charged. An allowable is an approved amount of reimbursement that the third-party payer decides the provider should receive for the services rendered to a patient. Because there is power in numbers, third-party payers are able to exact deep discounts from the full, or standard, charges of health care organizations and providers of care. The result is that those without insurance, including indigent patients, are charged at substantially higher rates for their health care. Some of these patients/clients have the ability to bargain for lower charges or settlement rates, but most do not have such leverage under our system.

EXERCISE 3-3

Discuss the following questions in class:
A) How would you determine a price for providing therapeutic exercise at an outpatient clinic using a market-based pricing strategy? How would you determine what is customary, prevailing, and reasonable?
B) What unit of measure for this service is most appropriate and why?
C) How would you determine a price for providing therapeutic exercise at an outpatient clinic using a cost-plus pricing strategy? Are there fixed, variable, or semivariable costs associated with providing this service?

Managerial Accounting and Financial Statements

Physical therapy managers can hire an accountant to provide reports about the economic activities and conditions of the physical therapy practice, but it is the manager's duty to make good decisions based on the information provided. A common practice of accounting is the periodic preparation of **financial statements** in accordance with generally accepted accounting principles (GAAP). This type of financial accounting information is typically used for reporting to those external to the business, such as stakeholders, shareholders, tax collectors (i.e., governmental agencies), and creditors. However, managers need to focus greater attention on **managerial accounting**, in which management reports are prepared in accordance with the needs of the practice and include objective measures of past operations and projected estimates for decision making about the future. In physical therapy practices, cost (i.e., a payment of cash in the present or future) is incurred for the purpose of generating revenue. Direct labor is the primary cost for providing physical therapy services, and indirect costs, sometimes referred to as *overhead*, comes from various sources, such as materials, equipment depreciation, consulting services, and so on. Revenue is the amount a practice earns by providing physical therapy services to patients/clients for a fee. Unfortunately, **assets** (i.e., resources owned by the business) or services are consumed in the process of generating revenue, creating expense. Although the terms *expense* and *cost* are often used synonymously, there is a slight distinction: Costs are incurred to generate revenue, and an **expense** is incurred through the generation of revenue. Physical therapy practice expenses are considered a cost of carrying out the physical therapy services because a business incurs the cost of practice expenses in order to generate revenue. Practice expenses can also be classified as direct expenses, such as clinical wages, medical supplies, and medical equipment, or as indirect expenses, such as administrative wages, office supplies, and all other expenses needed to run the practice. If revenues exceed expenses, the practice gains a **net income;** if expenses exceed revenues, the practice suffers a **net loss**.

There are four basic steps necessary for a physical therapist manager to gain an understanding of the financial workings of a practice. Learning the terminology is the first step to becoming a good manager of finances; therefore a general introduction to the language of finance is incorporated throughout this section. The second step is to understand the financial statements (e.g., **income statement**, **retained earnings statement**, **balance sheet**, statement of cash flow). The third step is to make decisions based on horizontal and **vertical analysis** of statements. The final step is to create a realistic **budget** for use in the next year or next several years.

Financial statements are reports prepared to summarize transactions that have taken place over a specified period of time (i.e., month or year). The first financial statement prepared is the income statement, which summarizes the revenues and expenses to highlight either a net income or a net loss for the period reported (Figure 3-2). In physical therapy practices, revenues are earned by providing services or selling DME. On the income statement, gross revenue is recorded under "fees earned."

[PT Practice Name] Income Statement For [Month/Year] Ending [Month/Date/Year]		
Fees earned:		
Services	$500,000	
Equipment sales	2,000	
Total operating revenue		$502,000
Operating expenses:		
Wage expense	$350,000	
Rent expense	2,500	
Supplies expense	500	
Equipment expense	50	
Miscellaneous expense	50	
Total operating expenses		$353,100
Net income		$148,900

FIGURE 3-2 | Sample income statement.

The net income or loss during the time period is reflected, respectively, as either an increase in **retained earnings** (i.e., **owner's equity**) or a decrease in retained earnings for the period. *Retained earnings* means the net income kept in possession of the company. These earnings are considered an asset of the owner or stockholders. Stockholders can receive a distribution of revenues called **dividends** from the gross revenues earned. Likewise, owners can withdraw their equity in the business as cash. The retained earnings statement is where net income is added to the retained earnings of the prior month or a net loss is subtracted from the retained earnings of the prior month. The retained earnings statement is affected by net income or loss and payments to stockholders or owners (Figure 3-3). Please note that the retained earnings statement links the income statement to the balance sheet. The net income or loss is taken from the income statement and recorded on the retained earnings statement; then, after calculations, the retained earnings is taken from the retained earnings statement and recorded on the balance sheet.

The balance sheet is a record of the physical therapy practice assets, liabilities, and the owner's or stockholders' equity for a given time period (Figure 3-4). Assets are material resources owned by or owed to the physical therapy practice (e.g., cash, accounts receivable, prepaid expenses, medical supplies, equipment, buildings, land).

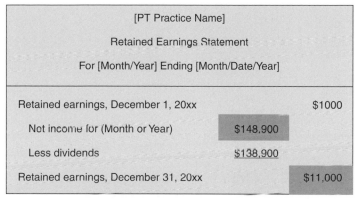

FIGURE 3-3 | Sample retained earnings statement.

Assets are listed on the balance sheet in the order of their difficulty to convert to cash (i.e., from easiest to the hardest). The importance of being able to quickly convert assets to cash will be addressed later in this chapter. **Liabilities** are debts owed to others outside the business (e.g., accounts payable, notes payable). Owner's equity, or stockholders' equity in corporations, is the money value or ownership rights of a party who holds interest in the business. When investors purchase shares of stock for part ownership in a company, the total amount of stock owned is called **capital stock**. Retained earnings are added to capital stock to gain a total of the owner's or stockholders' equity. Please note that adding the liabilities to the owner's equity will result in the equivalent sum of the business assets—hence the report title "balance sheet." Also note that cash, which is recorded under assets on the balance sheet, is the month or year ending cash on hand, which can be calculated through completing a **statement of cash flow** (Figure 3-5).

The statement of cash flow reports the cash transactions over a specific period of time (i.e., month or year). All cash transactions from operations activities, investing activities, and financing activities are recorded in the statement, and the year or month total should equal the amount reported for cash in the balance sheet.

The analysis of financial statements can provide important information for decision making. Financial statements can be analyzed by comparing items on a current statement with items on an earlier statement or by comparing individual items within a statement with other items in the same statement. In the analytical procedure known as **horizontal analysis**, items from the current statement are compared with statement items from a prior year or years. The income statement, balance sheet, and retained earnings statement often contain information that is interesting to compare with information from previous years. The comparisons are made by looking at the difference in items between years (i.e., gain or loss in the amount of the item) or by expressing the change as a percentage. For instance, cash on the balance sheet shown in Figure 3-4 is reported as $140,000. If this amount is compared with cash of $100,000 from last year's balance sheet, a difference of $40,000 is realized. Dividing the difference by the amount of the year past and

	[PT Practice Name]		
	Balance Sheet		
	For [Month/Year] Ending [Month/Date/Year]		

Assets		Liabilities	
Cash	$140,000	Accounts payable	$15,000
Supplies	15,000	Notes payable	80,000
Accounts receivable	11,000	Total liabilities	$95,000
Land	50,000		
		Stockholders' Equity	
		Capital stock	110,000
		Retained earnings	11,000	121,000
Total assets	$216,000	Total liabilities and stockholders' equity	$216,000

FIGURE 3-4 | Sample balance sheet.

multiplying that answer by 100 gives the percentage of change from one year to the next. For example:

40,000/100,000 × 100 = 40% increase in cash

Decision making for the next year is based on whether an increase or decrease in the item is preferable and the factors that affected the change for better or worse from a given year to the next. Similarly, vertical analysis compares difference scores and percentage of change; however, in vertical analysis the items under analysis are compared with the total within a single statement. For instance, it might be interesting to know what percentage of the total assets was cash. In our example, cash on the balance sheet was $140,000, and total assets were $216,000. Performing a percentage calculation reveals that cash is 64.8% of the total assets. So, the determination can be made that cash is the primary asset of the business. Relationships and trends can be assessed by vertical and horizontal analysis of financial statements. Expressing this comparison in both dollar and percentage amounts on the same statement can provide a useful means by which to make these comparisons. The word *comparative* is used in the title, before the name of the statement, to express that the document compares items across years. Both vertical and horizontal analysis can be represented on a comparative statement. A **common-size statement**, which expresses all items as percentages for ease of comparison, can be useful in comparing one physical therapy practice with another or with a practice standard or average.

Aside from the use of financial statements to assess the health of a physical therapy practice, the manager can use other analytical measures to assess the

[PT Practice Name] Statement of Cash Flows For [Month/Year] Ending [Month/Date/Year]		
Cash flows from operating activities:		
Cash received from patients/clients	$502,000	
Deduct cash payments for expenses and creditor payments	283,100	
Net cash flow from operating activities		$218,900
Cash flows from investing activities:		
Cash payments for acquisition of land		(50,000)
Cash flows from financing activities:		
Cash received from sale of stock	$110,000	
Deduct cash dividends	138,900	
Net cash flows from financing activities		(28,900)
Net cash flow and (insert ending month, date, year)		$140,000

FIGURE 3-5 | Sample cash flow statement.

practice's ability to meet financial obligations (i.e., solvency) and earn income (i.e., profitability).

Solvency measures, relevant to physical therapy practices, are used to assess the ability of the practice to pay long- and short-term debt (i.e., current and quick ratio, respectively), efficiently collect receivables (accounts receivable turnover and number of days' sales in receivables), and indicate the margin of safety to creditors (ratio of fixed assets to long-term liabilities and ratio of liabilities to stockholders' equity).

EXERCISE 3-4

A) Analyzing the current and quick ratios can provide useful information in comparison with previous periods or other physical therapy practice. Using the information from the financial statements in Figures 3-2 to 3-5 and the following formulas, determine the current and quick ratio.

Current Ratio = Current Assets/Current Liabilities

Quick Ratio = Cash + Assets Easily Converted to Cash/Current Liabilities

B) The ratio of fixed assets to long-term liabilities is particularly important to physical therapy private practices seeking to obtain loans. Fixed assets are relatively permanent and exist physically, such as buildings and equipment. Long-term liabilities do not come due for a period of longer than 1 year (e.g., notes payable). If the net fixed assets totaled $500,000 and the long-term liabilities totaled $100,000, what is the ratio of fixed assets to long-term liabilities?

C) Creditors and owners have claims against the total assets of the business. It is better for the owners to have a larger claim on the business assets than creditors because of the interest payments charged by the latter. Through the vertical analysis of the aforementioned balance sheet example, calculate the ratio of liabilities to stockholders' equity.

Ratio of Liabilities to Stockholders' Equity = Total Liabilities/Total Stockholders' Equity

Would you consider your finding to represent a large margin of safety? Why or why not? Comparing this ratio in a horizontal analysis can provide useful information to the practice.

Arguably, the most important solvency measures to a physical therapist manager are those that address efficiency in collecting receivables. Collecting receivables affects cash flow, which can determine whether the business is able to sustain itself. After providing and billing for a service, the physical therapist must await payment from the third-party payer, unless the patient/client paid in cash. Prompt collection of cash can be used to purchase assets or pay liabilities and stockholders. The longer the debt remains in accounts receivable (AR), the less likely it is that the practice will collect on the account. On the basis of monthly balances, the manager can calculate the AR turnover by dividing the net sales of services provided by the average net AR. Through horizontal analysis, the manager can assess the experience of an improvement or decline in the collection of receivables. The number of days' sales in receivables is the ratio computed by dividing the net accounts receivable at the end of the year by the average daily sales (calculated by dividing yearly sales by 365 days in a year). This estimate of the length of time that AR is outstanding provides an excellent indication of the efficiency of collection procedures and can be used in comparative analysis within the practice or as a comparison with other physical therapy practices.

Profitability measures assess the effectiveness and efficiency of the physical therapy practice in earning profit. The three primary measures used by physical therapy managers to assess profitability are the ratio of net sales to assets, the rate earned on total assets, and the rate earned on stockholders' equity. To assess the effective use of the practice assets, the manager can divide the net sales by the average total assets (excluding long-term investments) to calculate the ratio of net sales to assets. If two physical therapy practices have equal net assets, the practice providing the higher number of services is making better use of its assets. The rate earned on total assets takes into account the profitability of total assets regardless of whether the assets are financed by stockholders or creditors. By adding the interest expense to the net income and dividing the sum by the average total assets, a manager calculates the rate earned on total assets. The higher the rate earned on assets when compared with prior months or other businesses, the better the profitability of the practice. To focus on the rate of income earned on the amount invested by stockholders, the manager can divide the net income by the average total stockholder equity. This rate is typically higher than the rate earned on total assets because the interest paid to creditors is less than the amount earned on assets acquired with creditor's funding. The difference between the two rates is called *leverage*, and the greater the rate earned on stockholder equity compared with the rate earned on total assets, the better the leverage for the company. A comparison of these rates from year to year provides a good way to assess the profitability of the business.

The physical therapy manager needs to have instant access to financial information to continuously develop, maintain adequate control over, and effectively operate the practice. Practice management requires accurate financial information and good decision making, which can be assisted by being attentive to and using an effective budget. *Merriam-Webster's Collegiate Dictionary*[25] defines *budget* as "a statement of the financial position of an administration for a definite period of time based on estimates of expenditures during the period and proposals for financing them." A budget reflects knowledge of the financial situation of the business, with a projected plan for the future that incorporates specific goals and constant comparison with the actual financial results as they unfold. Budgets are usually developed for a fiscal year, but some managers may consider adopting a continuous budget, in which as one month closes, the corresponding budget for the same month of the following year is added, maintaining a 12-month projection into the future. Likewise, some managers may choose to start fresh each year without consideration of the prior year, a method known as *zero-based budgeting*. A more common approach is to project the next year's budget by revising the past budget in accordance with what actually took place during the year. This projection could encourage breaking even in the next fiscal year, improving productivity by setting a higher goal than the previous year, or breaking even in some areas and improving in others. Nonetheless, the budgetary goals should be specific, measurable, achievable, relevant, and timely. Setting budgetary goals too high (more stringent) can discourage employees, whereas allowing too much slack in a budget or budget line item by increasing the allotted amount of money available as a cushion can cause employees to spend the amounts remaining in the budget so as to prevent the budget from being cut in the next fiscal year.

Most physical therapy practices use a basic income statement format (Figure 3-6) for budgeting. The projected dollar amounts for each line item are placed in accordance with an income or expense account. Most computer-based budgeting programs will run reports with comparisons of the budget to actual income and expenses. A "profit and loss budget vs. actual" report lists the actual budget approved next to the current budget income or expenses. The columns in Figure 3-6 calculate the dollar amount over budget and the percentage of the budget used year-to-date. The reports can typically be customized to the physical

[PT Practice Name] 20xx Budget	
	Jan - Dec XX
Income	
Patient care services income	500,000.00
Annual conference income	4,000.00
Equipment sales income	7,500.00
Investment income	50,000.00
Total Income	561,500.00
Expense	
Wage expenses	350,000.00
Rent expense	30,000.00
Bank charges and fees	1,000.00
Continuing education expense	3,000.00
Donations	750.00
PT director expenses	6,600.00
Legal fees	18,000.00
Advertising expenses	9,000.00
Payroll taxes	70,000.00
Postage	1,000.00
Utilities expense	33,000.00
Miscellaneous expense	1,400.00
Total Expense	523,750.00
Net Income	37,750.00

FIGURE 3-6 | Sample budget.

therapy manager's needs and preferences. Some programs have graphing capabilities for a visual representation of the budget.

Budgets can be prepared for individual accounts or any combination of accounts on the income statement to address areas in need of developing, controlling, or directing (e.g., services, equipment, service expenses vs. administrative expenses). In lieu of budgets based on an income statement format, balance sheet budgets are also common. Balance sheet budgets developed specifically for cash receipts and payments or capital expenditures are frequently employed. Marketing budgets are also prevalent in physical therapy practices in settings throughout the PTCC.

EXERCISE 3-5

A) The four Ps of marketing (i.e., product, price, place, and promotion) are considered controllable variables that a physical therapy practice can use to generate an increased patient/client load.

 With regard to promotion, use the income statement format to develop a marketing budget that involves publicity, advertising, and personal selling for a physical therapy independent practice. Be creative in generating promotion strategies, and if internet access is available, develop a realistic understanding of the cost of each initiative. This activity may be performed in groups.

B) Create a personal budget using the following relevant categories:
Income: Monthly or yearly
Expenses: Housing (e.g., rent, mortgage, insurance, taxes, maintenance); Automobile (e.g., loan, insurance, gas, maintenance, plates, car wash); Food (e.g., groceries, dining out); Utilities (e.g., electric, gas, telephone, water/sewer, trash removal, cable, internet); Clothing; Child care; Donations; Health care (e.g., dental, eye care, insurance, prescriptions), Life or disability insurance; Savings; Taxes (e.g., federal, state, local, social security, real estate); Personal (e.g., shopping, gifts, furnishings, spending money); Education (e.g., loans, books, tuition, fees); Leisure (e.g., books/magazines, entertainment, sports, music, toys/games); Vacation; Legal expenses; Pet expenses; Credit card loans; Miscellaneous.

Departmental budgeting is an ongoing managerial process in which departmental or service needs are defined and developed, prioritized, reduced to final written form (proposal), submitted to administration, defended (as necessary), and approved. From payroll to supplies to capital expenditures to contingency outlays, departmental budgetary items must be carefully circumscribed and, once approved, appropriately employed. A budget allocation from administration becomes an appropriation from which monies may be spent over an operating period. Clinical managers may not exceed budgetary authorizations without approval from above. In public governmental organizations or systems, to exceed the budget without authorization may constitute a criminal violation of a state or federal antideficiency act. A "spend-it-or-lose-it" policy at the end of a fiscal year is a similarly inappropriate action for a financial fiduciary (e.g., a clinic manager in a position of trust).

Open-book management is a concept under which financial information within an organization (excluding individual employee compensation) is shared with employees throughout the organization on a need-to-know basis. It is a policy of few or no financial secrets. Similarly, input from key employees through a budgetary suggestion process is critically important to appropriately and efficiently acquire and utilize equipment and carry out parameters of business expansion. Figure 3-7 presents a sample employee input form showing capital expenditures and long-range facilities planning for a physical therapy clinic.

Employee Survey, Capital Budget Forecast, [PT Practice Name]

Jan. 10, 20xx

Dear Colleagues:

Please evaluate the proposed equipment, building, and related capital expenditures below and rank-order them for possible acquisition next fiscal year. Space is also provided to write-in proposals for additional capital expenditures. Thank you for your participation.

Avid Dollars, MBA, CPA

Chief Financial Officer

(PT Practice Name)

_____ 3-Dimensional Computerized Gait Analysis System

_____ Outpatient Clinic, Fulano de Tal Shopping Center Complex

_____ Surface EMG Unit

Write-in suggestion(s):

_____

_____

_____

FIGURE 3-7 | Employee survey, capital budget forecast.

SUMMARY

The PTCC model is useful in understanding the physical therapist's role in different health care settings and gaining a general understanding of site-specific reimbursement. Effective financial management and a thorough knowledge of site-specific reimbursement systems are essential to health care organizational survival. A physical therapist manager must gain an understanding of the financial workings of a practice through learning financial terminology, understanding financial statements, making decisions based on analysis of statements, and adhering to a realistic budget. Revenues and expenditures are the two principle components of financial statements. Key financial statements include the income statement, balance sheet, and statement of cash flow. Financial ratios allow decision makers to assess the financial "health" of an organization and include solvency measures and profitability measures. Budgetary management includes operational forecasting and administration of financial matters within a department, division, or organization. Open-book management involves all relevant parties in financial operational management of the organization.

REFERENCES AND READINGS

1. American Physical Therapy Association: *Code of ethics.* Available at: http://www.apta.org/AM/Template.cfm?Section=Ethics_and_Legal_Issues1& TEMPLATE=/CM/ContentDisplay.cfm&CONTENTID=21760. (Accessed March 3, 2007.)
2. American Physical Therapy Association: Guide to physical therapy practice (ed 2), *Physical Therapy* 81(1): s31-s42, 2001.
3. American Physical Therapy Association: *The reimbursement resource book*, Alexandria, Va, 2005, American Physical Therapy Association.
4. Bair J, Gray M, editors: *The occupational therapy manager*, Bethesda, Md, 1992, American Occupational Therapy Association.
5. Center for Medicare and Medicaid Services: U. S. Department of Health and Human Services. Retrieved at http://www.cms.hhs.gov/InpatientRehabFacPPS. September 10, 2006.
6. Cleverley WO: *Essentials of health care finance*, ed 4, Gaithersburg, Md, 1997, Aspen.
7. Coile RC: *The new governance: strategies for an era of health reform*, Ann Arbor, Mich, 1994, American College of Healthcare Executives.
8. Collins EGC, Devanna MA: *The portable MBA*, New York, 1990, John Wiley & Sons.
9. Copeland T: Cutting costs without drawing blood, *Harvard Business Review*, 78(5): 155-164, 2000.
10. *Current Procedural Terminology*, ed 4, Chicago, 1998, American Medical Association.
11. Curtis KA: *The physical therapist's guide to health care*, Thorofare, NJ, 1999, Slack, Inc.
12. Fearon HM, Levine SM: *1998 CPT & RBRVS update*, Alexandria, Va, 1998, American Physical Therapy Association.

13. Finkelman AW: *Managed care: a nursing perspective,* Upper Saddle River, NJ, 2001, Prentice-Hall.

14. Fowler FJ: Shutting down the rumor mill: HCFA proposed rule for PPS for acute rehabilitation, *Rehab Economics* 8(7): 78-82, 2000.

15. HCFA changes name, announces new initiatives, *Rehab Management* 14(6): 10, 2001.

16. Howatt G: Leading managed care plans never pay retail, *Star Tribune,* pp. D1, D8, Sept. 9, 2001.

17. *International classification of diseases-9-clinical modification,* Geneva, 1995, World Health Organization.

18. Jette DU, Grover L, Keck CP: A qualitative study of clinical decision making in recommending discharge placement from the acute setting, *Physical Therapy* 83(3): 224-236, 2003.

19. Kleinke JD: *Bleeding edge: the business of health care in the new century,* Gaithersburg, Md, 1998, Aspen.

20. Kovacek PR, Jakubiak K: *Managing physical rehabilitation in a managed care environment,* Harper Woods, Mich, 1998, Kovacek Management Services.

21. Longest BB, Jr.: *Health professionals in management,* Stamford, Conn, 1996, Appleton & Lange.

22. MacKinnon JM, Quillen S, Johnson JJ: Economic modeling as a component of physical therapy academic strategic planning, *Journal of Physical Therapy Education* 15(3): 25-31, 2001.

23. MacStravic S, Montrose G: *Managing health care demand,* Gaithersburg, Md, 1998, Aspen.

24. McDonnell K, Fronstin P: *EBRI health benefits databook,* Washington, DC, 1999, EBRI-ERF. The PDF can be found at http://www.ebri.org/publications/books/index.cfm?fa=hlthdb.

25. *Merriam-Webster's Collegiate Dictionary,* ed 11, Springfield, Mass, 2004, Merriam-Webster.

26. Murer C: Deciphering the details: an update on implementing PPS for inpatient rehabilitation facilities, *Rehab Management* 14(2): 24-25, 2001.

27. Nosse LJ, Friberg DG, Kovacek PR: *Managerial and supervisory principles for physical therapists,* Baltimore, 1999, Williams & Wilkins.

28. Privacy rule will force major changes in handling of patient information, *Health Lawyers News,* pp. 9-15, Feb 2001.

29. Private practice, part 2: clinical management, *Orthopaedic Physical Therapy Clinics of North America* 3(1), 1994.

30. Private Practice, part 1: office management, *Orthopaedic Physical Therapy Clinics of North America* 2(4), 1993.

31. Rasmussen B. *Reimbursement and fiscal management in rehabilitation,* Alexandria, Va, 1995, American Physical Therapy Association.

32. Stark I & II. 42 United States Code Section 1395nn.

33. Wachler AB, Avery PA: Stark II final rule—Phase I: a kinder and gentler stark? *Health Lawyer (Special Edition),* Chicago, Ill, 2001, American Bar Association Health Law Section.

34. Walter J: *Physical therapy management: an integrated science,* St Louis, 1993, Mosby.

35. Warren CS, Reeve JM, Fess WR: Financial and managerial accounting, ed 8, Mason, Ohio, 2005, Thomson South-Western.
36. Wilson CK, Porter O, Grady T: Leading the revolution in health care: advancing systems, igniting performance, ed 2, Gaithersburg, Md, 1999, Aspen.
37. www.cms.us.gov

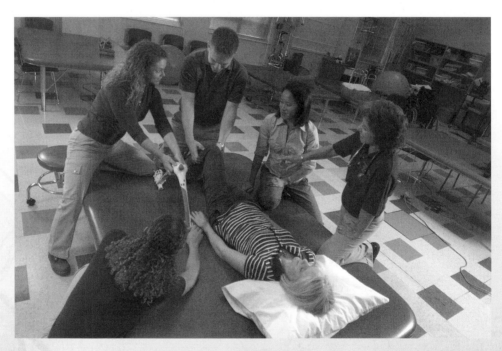

Courtesy University of Indianapolis.

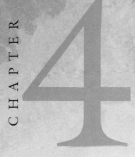

CHAPTER 4

Legal and Ethical Management Issues

Jonathan Cooperman

ABSTRACT

Physical therapist managers routinely encounter a variety of problems, many of which involve legal and ethical issues. Managers that rise through the ranks or have earned supervisory status through their clinical expertise or years of service are perhaps ill-equipped to recognize and deal with these issues. This chapter attempts to address the most common legal and ethical questions that confront physical therapist managers. Basic and applied ethics are discussed in addition to problems specific to the managed care milieu. Health care mal practice, sexual harassment, and employment law are reviewed, and these topics are followed by a discussion of federal laws that affect physical therapy practice.

KEY WORDS AND PHRASES

Abandonment
Affirmative defense
Age Discrimination in
  Employment Act of 1973
  (ADEA)
APTA *Code of Ethics*
APTA *Ethics and Judicial
  Committee*
APTA *Guide to Physical
  Therapist Practice*
APTA *Guide for
  Professional Conduct*
APTA *Standards of Ethical
  Conduct for the Physical
  Therapist Assistant*
Assault and battery
Beneficence
Breach of duty

Capitated contract
Causation
Civil Rights Act of 1964
Civil Rights Act of 1991
Compliance
Contract review
Covenant not to compete
Defamation
Deontological
Disability
Duty
Elder abuse
Employment at will
Employment law
Equal Employment
  Opportunities
  Commission (EEOC)
Essential function

Ethical behavior
Ethics
Expert testimony
Family Medical Leave Act
  (FMLA)
Fiduciary duty
Health care malpractice
Human resources
Independent contractors
Informed consent
Intentional conduct
Investigation
Managed care
Morals
Negligence
Negligent hiring
Noncompete clauses
Overutilization

Premises liability
Professionals
Qualified disability
Qui Tam
Reasonable
  accommodation

References
Risk management
Self-regulation
Sexual harassment
Sexual misconduct
Teleological

Title I of the Americans
  with Disabilities Act
  of 1990
Underutilization
Undue hardship
Wrongful termination

OBJECTIVES

1. Understand what is meant by the term *professional*.

2. Know the basic principles of health care ethics.

3. Appreciate that the APTA Code of Ethics guides ethical conduct for all physical therapists.

4. Recognize the key legal and ethical issues in managed care, and understand that the law and professional ethics have not changed substantially to accommodate the business of managed health care delivery.

5. Understand the nature of health care and physical therapy malpractice.

6. Formulate effective strategies to simultaneously optimize quality of patient care and minimize the risk of liability exposure in clinical practice.

7. Appreciate the legal and ethical aspects of patient informed consent.

8. Synthesize legal and ethical responsibilities and values into a formal patient informed consent policy statement in clinical physical therapy practice.

9. Understand how the law differentiates between negligence and intentional acts, and discuss their respective consequences.

10. Develop an understanding of the legal basis for sexual harassment in the health care workplace (including recent United States Supreme Court decisions), and structure appropriate risk management strategies to reduce the number of, and effectively deal with, those allegations.

11. Recognize some of the tenets of federal civil rights legislation, such as the Americans with Disabilities Acts (including recent United States Supreme Court decisions), and appreciate their impact on the health care workplace.

12. Possess a basic understanding of employment law issues.

INTRODUCTION

Physical therapist managers are faced with a number of challenges each day they arrive at the office. The formidable task of ensuring good practice is made more difficult still by the need to deal with a variety of legal issues. Those managers who do not work in large organizations and who do not have a **human resources** department to turn to find themselves involved in a dizzying array of legal issues, from **contract review** to **compliance** with federal regulatory schemes. Arguably more important is the fact that managers are responsible for setting the tone and establishing policies that lead to **ethical behavior** in the clinic.

Sometimes, it becomes quite difficult to separate one's legal and ethical responsibilities. Thomas H. Murray, Professor and Director of the Center for Biomedical Ethics, Case Western Reserve University made the following statement:

Rehabilitation **professionals**, like other health care professionals, work in an increasingly complex environment. What seemed obvious and easy a decade ago now may seem obscure and difficult. What are my ethical duties? What are my legal responsibilities? Called to a healing art, rehabilitation professionals have ethical and legal loyalties to their patients. These loyalties may be difficult at times to reconcile with organizational priorities, financial pressures, and personal needs or wants. Rehabilitation professionals, as with other health professionals, face complex and vexing problems. At times the problem may be mostly a matter of law with little ethical content. Most of the time, however, ethical and legal implications will be closely intertwined.[1]

Scott used a Venn diagram to demonstrate the overlap between law and **ethics** (Figure 4-1).[35] He also employs a four-quadrant grid (Figure 4-2) to focus on legal and ethical constructs and thereby guide clinical practice. It should be quite easy for the practitioner or student to provide practice examples that fall in the grids marked with two positives or two negatives. Good practice is both legal and ethical. In contrast, billing for services that were not performed would be an example of a behavior that is both illegal and unethical. However, it becomes more difficult to think of examples that fall in the grids with one positive and one negative. Occasionally, I am given the example of a physical therapist who breaks a law while claiming the infraction is for the good of the individual patient (e.g., treating a patient without a referral in a nondirect-access jurisdiction). In such a case, although it might be true that the patient ultimately benefits, it is also true that the clinician would violate the ethical principle of trustworthiness, which includes concepts of veracity and integrity.

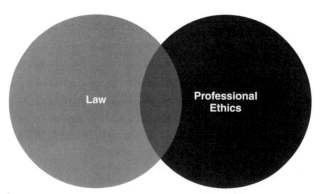

FIGURE 4-1 | Modern blending of law and professional ethics. (Courtesy Scott RW: *Professional ethics: a guide for rehabilitation professionals*, St Louis, 1998, Mosby, p. 10.)

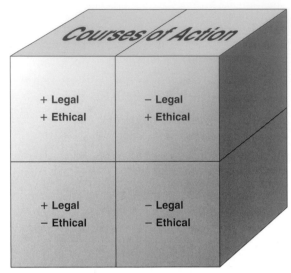

FIGURE 4-2 | Legal and ethical health care four-quadrant clinical practice grid. (Courtesy Scott RW: *Professional ethics: a guide for rehabilitation professionals,* St Louis, 1998, Mosby, p. 11.)

Similarly, if a clinician were to have a consensual sexual relationship with a patient, the clinician may admit that the conduct was unethical but (depending on where the practice is located) claim that no laws were violated, per se. However, many states incorporate the American Physical Therapy Association's Code of Ethics[2] in their state practice act—in essence, turning ethics into law. In such a case, unethical conduct is equivalent to illegal conduct.[5] Obviously, ethical dilemmas present many overlapping issues of law with many shades of gray.

This chapter provides an overview of some of the more common legal issues that will confront physical therapist managers. A discussion of basic ethical tenets and applied ethics is supplied to help managers guide their own behavior and the behavior of those for whom they are responsible. Case studies are used to clarify concepts and facilitate learning. The reader should realize that no two scenarios are ever exactly alike and that all legal and ethical problems should be handled on a case-by-case basis.

This chapter is intended to provide general legal information. Nothing in this chapter should be used in the place of legal counsel. All good managers have access to counsel and seek out professional legal guidance when appropriate.

ETHICS IN EVERYDAY PRACTICE

On Being a Professional and Self-Regulation

Physical therapists are now classified as professionals in all jurisdictions. Professions have historically demonstrated well-defined characteristics such as having a defined body of knowledge, formal education, and members who participate in research activities. Perhaps most important, professions demonstrate autonomy or self-governance. This includes the establishment of a Code of Ethics and **self-regulation**.

Wynia argued that defining a profession by its attributes is limiting and leads to a cynical view of the profession by society.[51] Wynia claimed, for example, that self-regulation, in the absence of an explicit moral base, is self-serving and insulates the profession from society. Instead, medical professionalism may be defined by its core elements: devotion to service (placing the goals of individuals and public health ahead of other goals), profession of values (speaking out about values), and negotiation within society (a social contract between physicians and the public). This argument could easily be extended to physical therapists or any other health care provider.

Physical therapists owe a special **duty** to their patients. Therapists act as a fiduciary, those in a special position of trust, toward their patients. This involves acting for someone else's benefit while subordinating one's personal interests to that of the other person (i.e., having the legal and ethical duty to act primarily in the patient's best interests). Wynia[51] spoke of the obligation of the professional and discusses the dangers of self-enforcement when it comes to professionals:

> In making a full case for professionalism, we do not wish to overstate the claim. In particular, we note that respect for human worth, trustworthiness, and the protection of important values are not the exclusive province of professionals; neither is competence. But they are particular obligations of professionals. We also remain mindful that professionals, no less than entrepreneurs or government officials, can misuse their power and have done so. The danger that power will be misused is inherent in any system that assigns authority to a group of people to police themselves. A full understanding of what professionalism entails provides some protection against this danger.

In spite of the potential flaws inherent in self-regulation, it remains a point of pride for professionals. The *Procedural Document on Disciplinary Action* of the American Physical Therapy Association guides the **Ethics and Judicial Committee** and the Chapter Ethics Committees when there are allegations of ethical wrongdoing.[28] The Association has taken great pains to attempt to ensure the rights of the complainant and respondent and to maintain confidentiality to the extent allowed by law.

Physical therapists would do well to stop and consider the ethical and societal responsibilities inherent in the label of professional. Too much emphasis has been placed on legal requirements and knowledge of federal regulations. True professionals focus on doing what is good and right for their patients.

Overview of Ethics

The basis for ethical conduct is our moral belief system. **Morals** are personal in nature and related to concepts of right and wrong. Morals arise from our society's beliefs, values, and principles. These beliefs were historically grounded in religion or specific cultures. However, more modern viewpoints recognize that in a democratic society, the state must answer to its citizens on equal terms *without* any underlying consideration to any particular religion or with the assumption that some persons' lives are inherently better than others.

Ethics can be described as a systematic analysis of morals and conduct,[30] that is, how individuals conduct themselves in their personal and professional endeavors. Ethics are often codified (i.e., collected and systematically arranged) into statements of conduct by professional organizations (i.e., codes of ethics). Although ethics are based on concepts of morality, their codification (and sanctions for a violation) sometimes resembles law. However, a code of ethics is merely an attempt to articulate the ideal conduct to which professionals aspire.

There are many classical ethical theories. These theories generally concern the actor, the specified conduct, or the consequences of that conduct. For example, **teleological** theory focuses on the consequences of conduct in an effort to determine whether or not the conduct was proper. In other words, the end would justify the means. Teleological theory involves the concept of utilitarianism—taking actions that promote the greatest social good, not necessarily actions that are good for a given individual. In contrast, **deontological** theory assesses conduct, which is to say that the means would justify the end.

Philosophers such as Aristotle focused on the actor and his or her virtues (moral goodness or excellence). Virtue-based ethicists tend to focus on the actor's character and judgment, not on the consequences of his or her conduct. Aristotle believed that virtues (and vices) are instilled by way of habit. Goodness leads to goodness!

The Code of Ethics

Physical therapist managers are seldom, if ever, academic ethicists. However, they are in the position of demonstrating ethical conduct and providing ethical guidance to those whom they manage. As noted earlier, physical therapy demonstrates autonomy or self-governance, which includes the establishment and enforcement of a code of ethics. In the profession of physical therapy, there is only one accepted *Code of Ethics*.[10] It is the product of the APTA's House of Delegates along with the companion *Standards of Ethical Conduct for the Physical Therapist Assistant* (see Appendix B).[38] Because this is the only code that has been articulated, it may therefore be argued that it is *the* code for physical therapy and therefore applicable to *all* physical therapists regardless of their association membership status.

APTA adopted a new *Code of Ethics* in 2000 (see Appendix A), in an effort to make the Code more patient-centered. Many states have incorporated APTA's *Code of Ethics* into their State Practice Act to varying degrees.[10] By doing so, the state license board is empowered to take action against a licensee who breaches the code but does not violate a law (see Figure 4-2). APTA also publishes *Guide for Professional Conduct* (see Appendix A) and *Guide for Conduct of the Affiliate Member* (see Appendix B),[10,38] which apply to physical therapists and physical therapist assistants, respectively. These documents are written to help individuals interpret the Code and the Standards and thereby guide conduct. They are intended to be much more dynamic documents than the more aspirational *Code* and *Standards*. These documents can and should be accessed and reviewed at www.apta.org.

Physical therapist managers should review and circulate these documents on a regular basis. An excellent exercise in solving ethical dilemmas is to create (or review) problems that fit into the various sections of the *Guide for Professional Conduct* and then have group discussions surrounding these issues. For example, imagine that a patient arrives at your clinic with a referral for poststroke physical therapy. Your clinic ordinarily does not treat patients with neurological impairments— you treat only patients with orthopedic problems. However, you have accepted a **capitated contract** from this patient's insurance company, and the patient insists that you are obligated to provide the therapy. To make matters worse, transportation is a significant problem for this patient and your clinic is within one block of his house—you are the only provider that the patient can get to. The APTA *Code of Ethics* states that physical therapists shall exercise sound professional judgment, and the *Guide for Professional Conduct* (paraphrased) states that if the problem is outside your expertise, you are obligated to refer the patient to an appropriate practitioner. You and your clinic now sit on the horns of a dilemma. Presenting this example or similar case studies during staff meetings or within an in-service fosters discussion that promotes ethical behavior. Moreover, good managers create an environment that encourages both staff and patients to report behavior they believe to be unethical. Although clinicians might consider reporting this type of behavior to their association's ethics committee or their state license board, it is much more desirable to have a complaint process in place within your organization. This encourages individuals to take responsibility for their actions and maintains open lines of communication.

Managed Care and the Ethical Dilemma of Limited Visits

The majority of Americans are now enrolled in some form of a **managed care** plan. Managed care, perhaps more correctly referred to as *managed payment*, reflects the attempt to control costs through various means. Controlling costs is a basic and accepted principle related to the business side of providing health care. In business the primary mission is to generate monetary profits, whereas in medicine the primary mission is to provide care. It is possible for these missions to co-exist. Unfortunately, however, some of the cost containment measures serve to detract from the practitioner-patient relationship.

It is interesting to note that in almost all business-related endeavors, the consumer is thought of as an asset. Within managed care, however, consumers of the product (i.e., the patients) are transformed into a liability the instant they begin to make use of the product. A managed care company will actually lose money if the customer/patient uses the service too much. Therefore managed care entities have structured financial incentives for the practitioner, who becomes an agent of the company. For example, physicians might be paid a bonus if they limit the number of referrals to specialists, thereby saving the managed care company money. This nonreferral for profit is antithetical to the ethical principle of **beneficence**.

In physical therapy, cost containment often comes in the form of a limitation in the number of patient visits allowed by the third-party payer. This is now true even for Medicare patients who have contracted with approved health maintenance organizations (HMOs). Many physical therapists, especially those in independent practice, deal with these externally imposed limits daily. Physical therapists, along with other health care practitioners, face a daily struggle to provide high-quality yet cost-effective care to their patients. When a patient is limited to only a few visits, therapists are immediately faced with several questions:

- Can I provide adequate care for the patient's problem within the allotted visit number?
- Am I ethically or legally obligated to treat the patient beyond the number of allowed visits?
- Can I request more visits, and will I receive them?
- Can I bill the patient directly for additional visits?

All health care providers have an ethical obligation to provide the best total care possible for their patients in all practice environments and under all payment systems. Founded in the ethical theory of beneficence (acting for the good of the patient), physical therapists act as a fiduciary for their patients. Patients understand that physical therapists will do what is best; thus patients and providers enter into a sacred relationship of trust.

When the decision to limit the number of visits allowed per incident (diagnosis) is made by someone other than the physical therapist before a physical therapy intervention, the physical therapist is confronted with the challenge of avoiding **underutilization**—providing fewer services than are warranted. This concern prompted the APTA 1997 House of Delegates to pass RC-33-97, which charged the Board of Directors (BOD) to address the issue. In turn, the BOD referred the task to the Ethics and Judicial Committee (formerly the Judicial Committee), which amended the *Guide for Professional Conduct* by adding a section that prohibits underutilization or **overutilization** of physical therapy services.

Ostensibly, this revision of the *Guide* was minimal in light of what is perceived as a significant problem in the profession. However, in an open letter to the membership printed in *Physical Therapy Magazine*, Ms. Charlene Portee, MS, PT, then Chair of the Ethics and Judicial Committee, wrote[29]:

> The Judicial Committee members worked diligently and considered several possible revisions to the *Guide*. We tried to provide a clear and uncomplicated way of reminding physical therapists of their ethical obligation to avoid underutilization. In the midst of an ever-changing health care arena, we cannot lose sight of our responsibility for maintaining and promoting ethical practice. We should always remain committed to providing the best total care possible for our consumer. Managed care has forced many physical therapists to limit the number of physical therapy visits that the patient receives. We should not allow our business arrangements to cloud our view of our ethical obligations. Section 3.3C of the *Guide* states that "when physical therapists judge that an individual will no longer benefit from their services, they shall so inform the individual receiving the services," thereby avoiding overutilization of physical therapy services. In turn, we have the same ethical obligation to safeguard the public from underutilization of physical therapy services. *As part of the obligation to safeguard the public from underutilization, physical therapists should inform their patients when*

they determine that the patient can benefit from physical therapy services, despite the exhaustion of third-party sources of payment." [italics for emphasis]

The following year, the Ethics and Judicial Committee once again amended the *Guide* Section 3.3(E) with even stronger language:

Physical therapists shall recognize that third-party payer contracts may limit, in one form or another, the provision of physical therapy services. Physical therapists shall inform patients of any known limitations. Third-party limitations do not absolve the physical therapist from adherence to ethical principles. Physical therapists shall avoid underutilization of their services.

It is worth noting that there are justifiable arguments set forth by third-party payers when they deny the request by physical therapists for more visits. One of the more cogent arguments is that the patient is often an employee who has chosen to work for a particular employer and may have bargained in good faith for their employment contract. That contract, whether express or implied, includes health care benefits. If the employer has chosen a particular health care plan on behalf of their employee, which limits the number of visits per condition or limits the time-frame for intervention, the third-party payer is under no obligation to exceed the limits of the policy. These arguments beg the question of how far a physical therapist must go in requesting more visits and if they are ethically obligated to provide them.

A purely ethical analysis reveals a rather straightforward response. Once a physical therapist has agreed to care for a patient, the therapist has an ethical obligation to provide appropriate care and act as a patient advocate to procure additional care. In other words, if a physical therapist knows that a patient requires more than the allotted number of visits, the therapist should find a way to provide them. Physical therapists, like other caregivers, have an ethical duty to protect the patient from harm and to do good for the patient. There is no doubt, however, that legal, business, and societal pressures complicate these decisions.

There is no legal requirement for a provider to extend care in the absence of payment. The *Guide for Professional Conduct* states only that a physical therapist shall render pro bono publico (reduced or no fee) services to patients lacking the ability to pay for services, as each physical therapist's practice permits.

However, physical therapists should be aware that the courts are beginning to closely scrutinize the actions of providers and payers for possible conflicts of interest. In an Illinois case, the court ruled that the plaintiff, Neade, could plead a cause of action for breach of **fiduciary duty** separate from a claim for medical **negligence**.[22] Neade's primary care physician (Dr. Portes) denied authorization for an angiogram that was recommended by another physician without first informing Neade that he had a financial incentive not to order additional tests. Neade suffered a massive myocardial infarction caused by coronary artery blockage and died. The court determined that the breach-of-fiduciary-duty claim was based on the defendant's failure to disclose to the plaintiff that he had a financial incentive to refrain from ordering any tests or referring Neade to a specialist to determine the cause of his symptoms. This case represents an example of a court-imposed ethical duty.

In a significant 2000 ruling, however, the United States Supreme Court in Pegram stated that incentive payments to health care practitioners by HMOs *do not* violate the fiduciary duty of HMOs.[27] The court went on to state that no HMO could survive without some incentive connecting physician reward with treatment rationing and that Congress had given its blessing to this form of health care delivery.[27]

In another example of ethical duty articulated and enforced by the courts, a physician suspected a deep vein thrombosis and wanted to extend his patient's hospital stay. His request was denied by the third-party payer, and the patient was discharged and later died as a result of thrombosis. In that case, the physician did not avail himself of the existing appeals process to extend the patient's stay. The Wickline court said that "the physician who complies without protest with the limitations imposed by a third-party payer, when his medical judgment dictates otherwise, cannot avoid his ultimate responsibility for his patient's care."[50]

In an attempt to describe the ideal physician-patient relationship, Emanual and Dubler created a construct of six Cs.[13] These are easily extended to the physical therapist. *Choice* refers to issues of **informed consent** and the ability of the patient to choose his or her provider or practice setting. *Competence* revolves around the practitioner's technical skill, clinical judgment, and current knowledge, as well the recognition of his or her own limitations. *Communication* is the ability to listen to the patient and to educate regarding the proposed intervention.* *Compassion* includes empathy and the ability to assist the patient in changing his or her perspective on the situation. *Continuity* means that the practitioner will develop a rapport with the patient and will commit to the care. Finally, an ideal relationship should have no *conflict* of interest.

For a few years after the Balanced Budget Act was passed, physical therapists noted an economic downturn, with the supply of therapists exceeding the demand and a concomitant decrease in salaries offered. Given the externally imposed limitation of treatment in a managed care environment, many physical therapists started to speak in terms of survival. In particular, therapists who accepted capitated contracts had to spread their resources across the number of patients covered in a particular geographic region in order to remain economically viable. Because of these circumstances, therapists were often forced to generate self-imposed limitations on the number of visits. It has been suggested that when a "survival ethos" is in place, ethical issues tend to be trivialized. Were physical therapists justifying unethical behavior (underutilization of services) by claiming it was for the greater good, because overall a greater numbers of patients could be served? In this example, the therapists would have been applying a utilitarian ethical theory to an ethical dilemma.

---

*It is the author's experience that a majority of patient complaints, whether legal, ethical, or administrative, are directly related to the practitioner's failure to communicate with either the patient or another health care provider. Timely, open, and honest communication is assuredly the best **risk management** tool that the physical therapist has at his or her disposal. With regard to managed care (or any payment) issues, therapists would do well to take time to discuss them with the patient before the intervention begins.

HEALTH CARE MALPRACTICE

Negligence

Negligence is a long-recognized legal concept in which liability is incurred because of conduct that fails to conform to an accepted standard. Negligence can involve an action or an omission. When a licensed medical care provider causes injury, the terms *professional negligence* or *medical malpractice* are used. Scott uses the term **health care malpractice** to account for the fact that plaintiff-patients (those bringing the lawsuit) may sue a variety of health care providers.[34] Historically, physical therapists were not sued as often as other care providers, especially when compared with physicians. This may be due to several reasons: (1) physical therapists did not have especially "deep pockets"; (2) physical therapists were viewed as caring providers and established strong rapport with their patients; and (3) physicians often controlled therapists, who were treated as technicians. In fact, in states where physical therapists were formerly classified as technicians and not as professionals, an action could be brought only under an ordinary negligence claim and not as malpractice (professional negligence). Times have changed! Physical therapists now carry substantial malpractice coverage and in our litigious society are just as likely to be sued as any other health care practitioner. The good news for physical therapist managers is that overall risk is still minimal. Consider that physical therapists can purchase malpractice insurance coverage of one million dollars per incident and three million dollars in the aggregate for approximately $300 or $400 per year. The low cost (compared with surgeons, who may pay as much as $50,000.00 to $150,000.00 per year) attests to the low risk of injury to patients. However, physical therapist managers must realize that risk does exist and that many physical therapists will become defendants in health care malpractice cases at some point in time.

CNA HealthPro recently released an analysis of physical therapist professional liability claims (with risk management recommendations) that occurred between December 1, 1993 and March 31, 2006. The average paid indemnity for all closed claims that included an indemnity payment (settlement or judgment) was $39,857.00. Among allegations with the highest frequencies were failure to supervise; injury during manipulation; improper technique; injury during heat therapy; and injury during resistance exercise or stretching.[9]

As with traditional negligence, the lawsuit may arise from an action or an omission. An act may be placing a patient's total hip replacement in a position of 120 degrees of flexion, internal rotation, and adduction, resulting in a dislocated hip; an example of an omission might be failing to secure a hemiplegic patient's shoulder in a sling after passive range of motion exercises, resulting in a dislocated shoulder. Health care malpractice must arise out of a medical claim. The patient who slips and falls while entering the locker room area will usually be able to bring suit only under a **premises liability** (ordinary negligence) theory. The different legal theories carry with them different statutes of limitations that are state-specific. In addition, malpractice actions generally require **expert testimony**, whereas ordinary negligence claims do not. When there is a controversy surrounding how the case should be filed, the court will decide. Both ordinary and professional negligence cases are civil actions, meaning that they are brought by private individuals who believe that they have been injured by the actions (or omissions) of the defendant(s). The remedy in almost all civil actions for negligence is money.

All health care malpractice cases have certain elements in common. In order to prevail, the plaintiff is obligated to prove the following:

- The defendant owed a duty of care.
- The defendant violated (breached) that duty.
- The defendant's (negligent) conduct caused the plaintiff's (patient's) injury.
- There was a compensable injury (i.e., monetary damages are required to compensate the patient).

A breakdown of each of the aforementioned elements will help the reader better understand health care malpractice.

Duty

The duty of care arises out of the special relationship physical therapists have with their patients. It is generally accepted that the duty attaches when the physical therapy intervention has begun. In the outpatient setting, physical therapists probably owe a full duty to the patient *after* the evaluation and, when informed consent is obtained, just prior to intervention.* This delay provides the therapist the discretion to determine whether the patient's problem falls within the therapist's scope of practice. In the inpatient setting, the duty may attach upon evaluation, depending on the facts of the case.

Breach of Duty

Physical therapists are held to a standard of care. Falling below that standard (i.e., offering substandard care) constitutes the **breach of duty**. The standard of care can be thought of as what an ordinary, reasonable physical therapist would do, given the same or similar circumstances. Although the particular facts of any claim of malpractice are always considered on a case-by-case basis, the most common way to determine the actual standard of care is through the use of expert testimony. Experts are almost always peers. In other words, another physical therapist is called on to testify as to the care provided by the defendant physical therapist. Scott reviewed the *Novey* case,[36] in which an appellate court remanded a case to the trial court after finding that an occupational therapist was *not* qualified to testify as to the physical therapy standard of care.†

---

*During the evaluation, therapists owe a limited duty—the duty to carry out the evaluation in a way that comports with professional standards.
†The Novey case may actually have been an exception to the majority standard requiring expert testimony by a peer. It could be successfully argued that there is sufficient overlap between "hand therapists," especially those who are certified (CHT), to allow an occupational therapist to testify about postoperative hand therapy, even when a physical therapist delivered the care.

Physical therapist managers should be especially aware of their own policies and procedures. When specific written policies and procedures or protocols are in place, nonadherence may be associated with significant liability. Employees are expected to unconditionally adhere to these procedures. If a lawsuit is filed, policies can be used as direct evidence to establish the standard of care. For example, if a postoperative total hip arthroplasty protocol states that the patient shall not be simultaneously placed in a position of hip flexion past 90 degrees and internal rotation, placing the patient in that position may be *prima facie* evidence of malpractice—that is, it is presumed true unless disproved by evidence to the contrary. Expert witnesses would simply be asked if the policies were reasonable and if, in fact, they were followed.

When deciding the standard of care, physical therapists should not fail to consider *The Guide to Physical Therapist Practice,* published by APTA.[16] This document includes preferred practice patterns, which describe relevant tests and measures as well as interventions appropriate to particular patient groups. It is based on expert consensus that provides boundaries of practice for specific patients. Therapists who offer treatment interventions that fall outside these boundaries must be prepared to justify their treatment techniques. Given the litigious nature of our society, it is probable that the justification for treatment will be requested during a deposition in the course of discovery in a medical malpractice lawsuit. In addition, because the *Guide* will be incorporated into all physical therapy practice, the preferred practice patterns may come to be viewed as *the* accepted standard of care.

Causation

The plaintiff in a malpractice case must also prove (by a preponderance or greater weight of the evidence) that the breach of duty caused his or her injury. Most courts require a showing of proximate, or a legal, cause. Proximate cause limits liability to injuries that were a *foreseeable consequence* of the acts of the defendant. In other words, the defendant would not be liable for harm that would be unforeseeable to the ordinary, reasonable person. This process is designed to protect the defendant from incurring liability for any injury that might have occurred but could not have been avoided.

Damages

The final element of proof in a health care malpractice claim is one of damages. The plaintiff must prove that a compensable injury occurred as a result of the defendant's negligence. For example, a physical therapist places a hot pack on the shoulder of his patient, a very thin older woman. The woman's shoulder is burned. If there were a first-degree burn, it would be difficult for the plaintiff/patient to claim significant damages, even though there was established duty, breach, and **causation**. However, if the same fact pattern is altered only so that the injury is a second-degree burn, which then became infected and eventually required a skin graft, damages would, understandably, be fairly easy to prove. It is interesting to note that many attorneys have commented that the only predictor of payment in malpractice cases is permanent **disability**, even in the absence of negligence.

In *Barvee v. Finerty*,[3] an Ohio Appellate court provided a definitive one-sentence summary of the elements of health care malpractice: "In order to establish medical negligence, plaintiff must establish, *through expert testimony*, standard of care recognized by [sic] medical community, failure of defendant to meet standard of care, and direct causal connection between negligent act and injury."

Regardless of the circumstances involved in any particular claim, there is rising evidence that an apology might go a long way toward decreasing potential risk. The American College of Physician Executives surveyed physicians and patients regarding their opinion on medical mistakes and how to deal with them. That survey revealed a growing consensus nationwide that honesty is the best policy when physicians and health care institutions err.[49a]

Informed Consent

Informed consent means providing a patient with information about a proposed treatment and its reasonable alternatives sufficient to allow the patient to make a knowing, intelligent, and unequivocal decision regarding whether to accept or reject the proposed treatment. A discussion on informed consent could easily be included within the section on professional ethics because this concept is founded on the ethical theory of autonomy: the patient's right to self-determination. Physical therapists are ethically bound to obtain informed consent before initiating any intervention. The *APTA Code of Ethics*, Principle 2 (*Patient Autonomy and Consent*) and especially section 2.4 A-E,[10] reflect the elements of informed consent. However, most jurisdictions now view the failure to obtain informed consent as malpractice. That means that claims alleging the plaintiff was harmed because of the failure to give consent to the treatment must comply with the applicable statute of limitations for malpractice actions and provide expert testimony as noted previously.

The common law (judge-made case law) elements of informed consent include:
- a description of the patient's problem *and* nature and purpose of proposed intervention
- risks associated with intervention (or nonintervention)
- reasonable alternatives to intervention
- benefits or prognosis associated with intervention

Physical therapist managers should take steps to ensure that the practice has a policy in place regarding informed consent. Although some clinics obtain written informed consent,* this approach has certain problems. Written forms tend to distance patients from their providers and can be overly broad or ambiguous. Patients must clearly understand what they are signing. Health care practitioners

---

*This generally involves having the patient sign a standard form listing the aforementioned elements and confirming that he or she consents to the proposed intervention.

should realize that written forms do not absolve them of liability. Moreover, unless the claim of malpractice is clearly based on the lack of informed consent, having obtained informed consent is *not* a defense against a claim of malpractice. In addition, each modality and treatment protocol would require separate consent, and possibly separate forms. Physical therapists should also keep in mind that the consent to treat frequently signed by patients is *not* the same as informed consent because the patient has not been informed of anything. Physical therapists may, however, choose to employ written forms when performing procedures with a higher risk of injury (e.g., cervical manipulation).

Informed consent may be obtained orally, whether it is stated expressly or implied from the surroundings. However, proof of oral consent is more difficult and could be demonstrated only through the testimony of witnesses. One alternative to obtaining written informed consent is to have a policy that states all providers will obtain informed consent and to continually review that policy with physical therapists on staff (see inset).

Informed Consent Policy Exemplar

Subject: Informed Consent
Effective Date:
Policy: All licensed practitioners shall obtain informed consent before beginning a physical therapy intervention.
Purpose: Obtaining informed consent ensures that the patient has made a knowing, intelligent, and unequivocal decision regarding physical therapy intervention.
Procedure: Physical therapists and other licensed practitioners at XYZ Rehabilitation Center *shall* obtain patient informed consent before beginning any intervention. This may be done orally, provided the practitioner uses language understandable to the patient and provided the patient demonstrates adequate understanding of informed consent. Elements of informed consent shall include, but are not limited to, disclosure of the following:

- The nature of the proposed intervention
- Material risks of harm or complications
- Reasonable alternatives to the proposed intervention, and
- Goals of treatment

Informed consent shall be documented in the patient's chart.

All physical therapists struggle with the issue of obtaining informed consent from the confused, incoherent, or globally aphasic nursing home patient who has not been adjudicated as incompetent (lacking the legal capacity to make decisions). Physical therapists must use their discretion and act in a professional manner when treating these patients. With regard to minors and others who have court-appointed guardians, it is the legal and ethical obligation of the physical therapist to obtain consent from the parent or guardian before intervening.

It is important for the physical therapist manager to realize that, from a legal standpoint, few if any allegations of malpractice are ever based on the failure to obtain informed consent. Rather than focusing on the legal aspect of informed consent, managers may do well to consider that informed consent is a back-and-forth communicative process with their patients. This approach fosters ethical interventions and at the same time makes the patient an active participant in the rehabilitation process. Having patients take an active role in their care is good practice and a good risk management strategy. The most common basis for all complaints—administrative, ethical, and legal—is a lack of communication (or miscommunication) between patient and provider. For example, a physical therapist who explains in detail why he or she is palpating the pubic tubercles during an examination (including, perhaps, having the patient self-palpate or view an anatomical model) would understandably incur much less risk of an allegation of **sexual misconduct** than the therapist who simply proceeds to palpate. Physical therapist managers should conduct in-services to review strategies for improved communication.

Abandonment

A concept related to informed consent is that of **abandonment**. *Abandonment* may be defined as the unilateral and inappropriate termination of a physical therapist-patient relationship. Physical therapists should always be cognizant of the fact that abandonment is more or less a one-way street. Patients may unilaterally terminate their care at any time, whereas health care practitioners have a duty not to walk away from the patient. It should be noted, however, that there has never been a reported case of negligent abandonment against a physical therapist. Reasons to terminate care might include failure to pay for services rendered or an irreconcilable personality conflict between the patient and the physical therapist. Certainly, achieving treatment goals or reaching maximal medical improvement would also justify terminating care. The law does not obligate a physical therapist to continue to treat a patient who needs further treatment but only to give adequate advance notice of the intent to terminate the care. Substitute physical therapists (e.g., during vacation, after employee termination) do not generally support claims of abandonment. Managers can avoid abandonment claims by adopting written policies related to no-shows and the use of substitute providers.

CASE STUDY 4-1

Mary, a physical therapist, works part-time in the home health setting and is employed by the local community hospital. She treats only patients with total joint replacements. Mary receives a referral for Elizabeth, a pleasant 78-year-old woman who recently underwent a total knee arthroplasty. Mary performs a detailed examination and sets up an appropriate plan of care, which concentrates on activities of daily living (ADLs), strengthening, and gait training. As the weeks progress, Elizabeth becomes independent in ADLs and progresses from ambulating with a walker to a cane. In fact, she becomes independent with the cane on level surfaces. Mary adjusts the plan to focus on stair climbing—the last functional goal

CASE STUDY 4-1

to achieve before Elizabeth can be discharged. On Wednesday, Mary goes to Elizabeth's apartment at the appointed time. She asks Elizabeth how things are going and proceeds to walk alongside of her in the apartment. They walk toward the stairwell of the apartment house so that Mary can help Elizabeth work on stair climbing. However, just as they pass through the doorway of Elizabeth's apartment into the hallway, Elizabeth trips and falls. It is obvious to Mary that Elizabeth has fractured her femur. Mary stabilizes Elizabeth and calls for help. The paramedics transport her without incident to the local hospital, where surgery is required to fixate the fracture. Unfortunately, Elizabeth's wound becomes infected, and eventually she is diagnosed with gangrene. Her leg is amputated above the knee. Mary feels terrible about the turn of events—and even worse when she is served with notice that both she and the hospital/employer are being sued for malpractice. The suit alleges that Mary breached the standard of care when she allowed Elizabeth to ambulate without a gait belt (it was in Mary's hand but not around Elizabeth when the incident occurred) and allowed her to fall. The suit alleges that it was foreseeable that not using a gait belt would create a higher risk of falls and that the fall proximately caused the fracture. In this case, the hospital policy on the use of gait belts clearly speaks to the discretion of the physical therapist.

DISCUSSION OF CASE STUDY 4-1

Does Mary have a defense to this claim? Did she in fact commit malpractice? In this scenario, it is obvious that Mary owed a duty of care to Elizabeth and that the fall proximately caused the injury. It could easily be argued that a gait belt would have prevented the fall. However, this case really turns on whether Mary acted as a reasonable, ordinary physical therapist would have under the same or similar conditions. *Should Mary have used a gait belt?* Mary had already established that Elizabeth was independent with a cane on level surfaces and had documented her status. The gait belt was required for stair climbing only. Expert testimony would, one might hope, establish that a physical therapist would have employed the gait belt only when working on stair climbing. The plaintiff's situation is regrettable, but the plaintiff was not successful in her malpractice claim against Mary and the hospital. (Note that policies and procedures for the use of gait belts should always refer to their use at the discretion of the physical therapist.)

Liability for Intentional Conduct

Negligence may be described as actionable carelessness. **Intentional conduct**, in contrast, includes affirmative acts. Although many types of conduct could be categorized as intentional,* this chapter focuses on **assault and battery**, **elder abuse**, and sexual misconduct.

---

*Intentional torts may cross a number of legal specialties, including business law, criminal law, and health care law. For a more complete discussion on intentional conduct, the reader is directed to Chapter 3 of Scott RW: *Promoting Legal Awareness in Physical and Occupational Therapy*, St Louis, 1996, Mosby.[36]

Assault and Battery

The terms *assault* and *battery* are commonly used in concert but have distinct legal definitions. An assault is a willful attempt or threat to inflict injury on another when coupled with an apparent ability to do so. An assault may be committed without actual physical contact. In some jurisdictions, there are further classifications, such as simple assault and assault with a deadly weapon. Battery, on the other hand, is intentional conduct that requires some physical contact (e.g., injury or offensive touching). All states have criminal laws dealing with assault and battery, but it can also be a tort (civil wrong for which an individual citizen could sue). If, for example, a male physical therapist made a pass at a female patient and reached across the plinth to grab her, his actions would constitute an assault. If he succeeded in his efforts and touched her breast, his actions would constitute battery. Consent is an absolute defense to assault and battery, reinforcing the view of informed consent as a risk management measure. The example provided is appropriate to the health care milieu, especially given that claims of sexual misconduct are on the rise.

A sexual assault is commonly defined as a nonconsensual touching of a patient for the purpose of arousing or gratifying the sexual desires of either party to the relationship. Sexual abuse is often thought of as engaging in sexual conduct with an individual who is incapacitated or to whom the perpetrator owes a special duty of care (e.g., minors, students, the elderly). Sexual abuse includes fondling, touching, sexual threats, sexually inappropriate remarks, and any sexual activity that the other party is unable to understand or unwilling to consent to or is threatened or physically forced into doing. Either definition (assault or abuse) can apply in patient care. In fact, many state statutes do not distinguish between the two.

Elder Abuse

Physical therapists have historically served the elder population, and America is aging rapidly. Approximately 13% of Americans were 65 and older in 1990 as opposed to 11% in 1980, making this group the fastest growing segment of the United States' population. Today there are more than 1.5 million people living in 20,000 nursing homes in the United States. Unfortunately, that demographic shift means that society has to deal with an increasing number of cases of elder abuse, as well as the issues of confinement and neglect. *Elder abuse* can be defined as the infliction of physical pain or injury on an older person. It can include the improper use of restraints.*

Emotional abuse includes verbal assault (i.e., threat to inflict harm, coupled with an apparent ability to do so), threats of maltreatment, harassment, and intimidation intended to compel the elderly person to engage in activity from which they have

---

*For a detailed discussion of physical restraint issues, the reader is directed to Cooperman JM, Scott RW: Physical restraint: legal and risk management issues, *Physical Therapy Magazine*, July 1998, pp. 58-61.

BOX **4-1** ■ **Characterizations of Elder Abuse**

- Physical and sexual abuse: active physical
- Verbal assaults: active emotional
- Confinement or denial of privileges: passive physical
- Absence of love and caring/any attempt to dehumanize: passive emotional

a right to abstain or to refrain from conduct that they have a right to enjoy. Neglect is the failure to provide, or the willful withholding of, the necessities of life, including, but not limited to, food, clothing, shelter, or medical care. *Confinement* means restraining or isolating an older person for nonmedical reasons. In fact, the definition of *elder abuse* has been broadened to include emotional and financial as well as physical abuse (Box 4-1).

Regardless of the characterization, and despite well-intentioned federal regulations and similar state statutes, most elder abuse is not reported. Underreporting has been estimated at 90%.

The physical therapist manager should be familiar with mandatory reporting requirements that currently exist in 43 states and the District of Columbia. Generally, health care and social service workers are named in the reporting statutes. For example, although physical therapists are not directly named in Ohio's reporting statute, the state statute includes the following language: "any senior service provider" (those who provide care to the elderly), and any employee of any hospital, nursing home, residential care facility, home for the aging, peace officer, clergy, ... having reasonable cause to believe that an adult is being abused, neglected or exploited, or is in a condition as a result of abuse, neglect, or exploitation *shall immediately report* such belief to the county department of human services." The statute goes on to state that any person reporting shall be immune from civil or criminal liability resulting from such **investigation** except liability for perjury, unless the person has acted in bad faith or with a malicious purpose.

Consensual Sexual Relations With Patients and Sexual Harassment

Because of the nature of the intervention (i.e., private and requiring hand-on treatment), physical therapists may be at a greater risk for allegations of sexual misconduct or **sexual harassment** than other health care providers. In fact, the incidence of sexual misconduct has long been disproportionately high in the health care environment. *Only* an allegation of sexual misconduct or harassment would be sufficient to create significant problems for a physical therapist. State license boards, association ethics committees, and local prosecutors generally take these allegations very seriously. In addition, the defendant-provider is always at risk for a civil lawsuit. Physical therapist managers must be aware of current sexual harassment law to create and enforce appropriate policies. All providers should be aware that professional liability polices do not usually provide coverage for these type of claims. This section provides general information on consensual relations with patients and sexual harassment; it is also meant to inform the reader of the recent United State Supreme Court cases and how they affect the responsibilities of managers and agents of the employer. As always, risk management is key in lessening the chance that these claims will be brought.

The topic of sexual harassment often emerges in discussions of **employment law**. Because of its prevalence in the health care workplace, it is included here in a separate section. Unlike some of the more esoteric legal concepts associated with employment law, this topic can and should be broached and managed by nonlawyers.

Consensual Relations

Consensual relations with a patient are not possible. Because of the fiduciary duty physical therapists owe to their patients, the issue of consent is a fiction. Under no circumstances can there be a consensual relationship given the vulnerability of the patient and the power that the therapist holds over him or her. Therefore the use of the term *consensual* becomes meaningless. The physical therapist is always responsible for creating the relationship, regardless of who might have initiated the emotional or physical contact. APTA's *Guide for Professional Conduct* states unequivocally that physical therapists "shall not engage in any sexual relationship or activity, whether consensual or nonconsensual, with any patient while a physical therapist/patient relationship exists."[10] *The Guide for Professional Conduct* fails to provide direction or guidance for physical therapists who find themselves involved in a nontherapeutic relationship with one of their patients. There is no denying that physical therapists engage in this type of behavior. The leaders of the profession must continually educate therapists as to the inappropriateness of this type of conduct. However, physical therapists who find themselves involved with a patient should (1) immediately disengage themselves from the care of that patient and (2) transfer the patient's care to another provider.

Sexual Harassment

In the past 30 years, the United States has passed significant federal legislation related to sexual harassment. Unfortunately, our government leaders have produced a rather nefarious public history. The claims of sexual harassment against then Supreme Court nominee Clarence Thomas in 1991 brought this issue to national attention. Although Justice Thomas was eventually cleared of the allegations, the case drew public attention to workplace behavior. In 1992, the U.S. Navy was embroiled in the so-called Tailhook scandal when female naval officers attending an aviators' association convention were forced to run through a gauntlet in a hotel corridor. U.S. citizens have also witnessed the resignation of two members of Congress after accusations of sexual misconduct.* Paula Jones accused President

——
*Bob Packwood, U.S. Senator from Oregon, resigned in 1994, and Mel Reynolds, a U.S. Representative from Illinois, resigned in 1995.

William Jefferson Clinton of sexual harassment that allegedly occurred during his tenure as governor of Arkansas. Despite these high-profile cases, the number of cases filed each year (13,136 in 2004 and 12,679 in 2005) suggests that the average American does not seem to fully grasp the concept of appropriate behavior in the workplace or the consequences of inappropriate behavior.

Title VII of the 1964 Civil Rights Act forbids discrimination against employees (and job applicants) on the basis of race, gender, religion, and national origin. Title VII cases specifically apply to employment-related discrimination. Although Title VII cases apply only to employers with 15 or more employees, several state laws mirror Title VII and allow relief for individuals who work in smaller companies. Those receiving federal funds (e.g., employees in the public school systems) can file claims of sexual discrimination under Title IX of the Education Amendments of 1972.

The **Equal Employment Opportunities Commission** (EEOC)—the federal regulatory body charged with interpreting and enforcing these laws—states that sexual harassment is a form of sex discrimination that violates Title VII. In 1981, the EEOC promulgated its guidelines defining sexual harassment[37]:

Unwelcome sexual advances, requests for sexual favors, and other verbal or physical conduct of a sexual nature constitutes sexual harassment when any of the following apply:

1. Submission to such conduct is made either explicitly or implicitly a term or condition of an individual's employment
2. Submission to or rejection of such conduct by an individual is used as the basis for employment decisions affecting such individual.
3. Such conduct has the purpose or effect of unreasonably interfering with an individual's work performance or creating an intimidating, hostile, or offensive working environment.

The types of conduct that might be considered sexual harassment include, but are not limited to, epithets; slurs; negative stereotyping; or threatening, intimidating, or hostile acts. A closer analysis of the EEOC guidelines reveals that there are two categories: adverse employment decisions and hostile environment. Adverse employment decisions (firing, demoting, transferring, denying promotion, and denying raises) are sometimes referred to as *quid pro quo*, a Latin term meaning "something for something." In contrast, most of the cases brought before the EEOC deal with allegations of a hostile or offensive work environment. In each case the Commission will look at the record as a whole and at the totality of the circumstances. All complaints are decided on a case-by-case basis. Recently, the Supreme Court has provided a somewhat different approach as discussed in cases to follow.

Regardless of the way the case is viewed, the complaints must allege that the conduct is unwelcome, is of a sexual nature, and unreasonably interferes with the work environment. The harasser may be a man or a woman, a supervisor, an agent of the employer, a co-worker, or a non-employee. The hostile environment may manifest itself in a one-time incident of sufficient severity; however, a one-time incident will generally involve physical contact in order to be actionable.

A common misconception is that the law protects harassment not related to gender or other protected classes (e.g., race, religion, ethnicity). In fact, harassing conduct not related to gender is *not* actionable under a Title VII claim. An Ohio Appellate Court articulated this concept[20]:

> The justice system cannot be the arbiter of feelings hurt and egos bruised as a result of mere insensitive and tasteless statements made by an individual in a position of authority.

Of course, this does not mean that managers should tolerate bad behavior. Rather, it means that there is no available federal venue for complaint related to generic harassment. Physical therapist managers should encourage mutual respect among all employees.

Studies have spoken to the prevalence of sexual harassment in the physical therapy workplace. In a national survey of physical therapists, DeMayo found that 86% of the respondents reported having experienced some form of patient sexual behavior in the course of practice, with the vast majority not rated as harassment. However, 67% reported at least one incident of sexual harassment. Triezenberg assembled a panel of experts to identify current ethical issues facing physical therapists.[46] Identification and prevention of sexual misconduct was a consensus choice among the panelists.

In 1996, Lake Research conducted an APTA-commissioned survey on sexual harassment. Although few of the respondents initially chose sexual harassment as a major problem (they cited managed care), 18% believed they had personally experienced harassment. Moreover, after hearing a number of inappropriate sexual behaviors, 37% stated they had experienced at least one of those behaviors. Suggestive and crude remarks and sexual jokes and stories are the most common forms of harassment, which, the survey found overwhelmingly, occurred at work. Hospitals were listed as the most troubling setting. Those who responded to the survey noted that patients were overwhelmingly the worst perpetrators. Few respondents indicated that they had reported episodes of harassment to the authorities. The most common reactions to harassment are talking to the perpetrator; talking to co-workers, family, and friends; and doing nothing.

The 1998 Supreme Court Cases

In 1998, the U.S. Supreme Court decided several cases involving sexual harassment issues. Before this time, the Supreme Court had issued only two decisions (in 1986 and 1993) related to sexual harassment. *Oncale v. Sundowner Offshore Enterprises, Inc.*, involves a male roustabout on a Louisiana oil rig who was subjected to sex-related and humiliating actions by the other male members of the crew.[26] In this case, the Court ruled unequivocally that same-gender sexual harassment is actionable under Title VII. Although firm in its ruling that same-gender sexual harassment can exist, the Court seemed to go to great lengths to avoid the creation of a sterile workplace:

> The real social impact of workplace behavior depends on a constellation of surrounding circumstances, expectations and relationships which are not fully captured by a simple

recitation of the words used or the physical acts performed. Common sense, and an appropriate sensitivity to social context, will enable courts and juries to distinguish between simple teasing or roughhousing among members of the same sex, and conduct which a reasonable person in the plaintiff's position would find severely hostile or abusive.*

More significantly, in two combined cases the Court clarified the responsibilities of the employer for the acts of its agents, supervisors, and managers. In *Ellerth v. Burlington Industries*,[12] the court reviewed the case of a woman (Ellerth) who had been sexually harassed by a midlevel manager who threatened her position with the company. However, Ellerth received her promotions and, as such, suffered no "tangible job detriment," the language now preferred by the court. It should also be noted that Burlington had an internal sexual harassment complaint procedure that Ellerth failed to take advantage of. The Supreme Court applied principles of agency law and stated that the plaintiff will prevail if he or she can show the following: (1) that the harasser spoke on behalf of the employer and the plaintiff relied on this apparent authority or (2) that the harasser was able to harass the plaintiff because of the existence of a supervisory relationship. If the plaintiff/employee is successful in proving any of these points, then the employer is liable. However, the Supreme Court reserved an **affirmative defense** for the employer. If the employer can prove two points, the employer will escape liability:

- The employer exercised reasonable care to prevent and correct sexual harassment.
- The plaintiff unreasonably failed to follow the sexual harassment complaint procedure published by the employer.[†]

In *Farragher v. Boca Raton*, a case decided along with Ellerth, the Supreme Court stated that the city of Boca Raton could not utilize this affirmative defense because it failed to disseminate its sexual harassment policy to all municipal employees.[14] The aforementioned affirmative defense is available to the employer only when the plaintiff has suffered no tangible job detriment, as in Ellerth's case. If, in fact, the plaintiff has suffered tangible job detriment, then the employer is strictly liable (i.e., no defense is available). Regardless, it is very important for managers to realize that the employer is clearly subject to vicarious liability for acts of supervisors who create a hostile environment.

With regard to allegations of co-worker sexual harassment or complaints about the conduct of visitors (e.g., vendors) to the clinic, the courts apply a negligence standard. In other words, the employer is liable for the conduct of others if it can be proven that the employer knew, or should have known, about the alleged harassment.

---

*Author's opinion.
†Simply having or adopting a written policy is not enough. The policy must be communicated to all employees. Most employers include their sexual harassment policy in the employee handbook.

PRACTICAL CONSIDERATIONS AND PRACTICE-BUILDING BEHAVIOR

All employees working within a physical therapy environment must be aware that their conversations and actions might offend patients, other health care providers, and visitors to the clinic. Therapists need to respect the fact that comments casually made might be acceptable to their intended recipient but might, at the same time, offend someone else. For example, the physical therapist who makes an offhand and ribald comment to another therapist might be unaware that an aide was within earshot. If those inappropriate comments offended the aide, and they were the type of comments that would offend a reasonable person in a similar situation, then the aide could bring a complaint of sexual harassment.

Access to the Internet and electronic mail pose additional problems for the physical therapist manager. Everyone who has access to the Internet or email should be cognizant of what is being sent and received. Sexually charged jokes, explicit pictures, and personal comments do not belong in the workplace, even if the sender assumes that they are being sent through secure channels.

Rather than deciding to live and work in a sterile environment, physical therapists must take responsibility for their actions and show respect for others. Physical therapist managers should develop a zero-tolerance policy when it comes to telling inappropriate jokes and engaging in sexual repartee or innuendo. All providers should ensure that conversations stay on a professional level.

Dealing With Complaints

All physical therapy practices, large and small alike, should have a formal written sexual harassment policy in place. This policy typically is located in the employee handbook or the policies and procedures manual (or both places). An example of a sexual harassment policy is found in Appendix C. This policy was adapted from a sample policy created by the Ohio State Bar Association for Ohio law firms. Physical therapist managers can use this policy as a template for their own practices.

Investigating Allegations of Sexual Misconduct

Allegations of sexual misconduct or harassment can have a chilling effect on any institution or business, including a physical therapy practice. Many managers and supervisors will listen to the complaint and then attempt to either placate the complainant or minimize the alleged behavior. Dealing with these types of complaints may be personally disturbing, but it is vital to the employer-employee relationship and the overall success of the business. A prompt investigation of the alleged improprieties demonstrates that management takes these types of complaints seriously. Prompt and complete investigations also promote a quick resolution. Complaints that surface months and years later are difficult, if not impossible, to investigate. Delayed investigations of current complaints produce the same results.

As previously noted, the investigation should be undertaken promptly—usually within 2 or 3 days. The investigator can be a supervisor, manager, human resources employee, or a third party with no connection to the business. As a general rule, more than one individual within a practice should be designated to take complaints. The investigator should assure employees that confidentiality will be protected to the extent possible, while noting that, at some point in time, the respondent will have the right to face their accuser. At a minimum, the investigator must interview the complainant and the respondent. The investigator should make every effort to identify and interview witnesses as well. By asking the complainant to write down everything that occurred, the investigator will not only document the complainant's version of events but also help the complainant achieve catharsis. The report of the investigator should be dated and signed by the complainant and then reviewed and signed by witnesses.

The employer should encourage employees to report any harassment to management *before* it becomes severe or pervasive. Even in the absence of complaints, managers should take every step possible to correct behavioral deficiencies. The sexual harassment policy should make it clear that the employer will tolerate neither harassing behavior nor retaliation against those who complain or participate in an investigation.

RISK MANAGEMENT

The box below lists several risk management tips for physical therapist managers. One of the simplest and most effective risk management strategies is obtaining informed consent. Patients who are being touched need to consent to that touch. Therapists using techniques that involve therapeutic touch on an area away from that of the chief complaint should take extra time to explain their approach, eliminating any potential misunderstandings that might arise.

Risk Management Tips

- Adopt a knock-and-enter policy.
- Require same-gender chaperone.
- Have a written policy statement in place defining sexual harassment.
- Take steps to educate the workplace about sexual harassment.
- Express strong disapproval of inappropriate behavior.
- Have a grievance procedure in place, and communicate it to employees.
- Conduct immediate, fair, unbiased investigations after an allegation of sexual harassment.
- Take prompt remedial action when inappropriate conduct is identified.*
- Establish a sexual harassment policy, publish it, and communicate it to all employees.

---

*The EEOC recognizes prompt and remedial action as an appropriate defense to claims of hostile workplace. This is not true for claims of quid pro quo (in which the harassment is an explicit or implicit condition of employment or is used as a basis for employment decisions).

CASE STUDY 4-2

John, a single male therapist who is 28 years old, evaluates Barbara, a 26-year-old female. During the course of the evaluation, John inquires about Barbara's stress level and learns that she is separated from her husband and is going through divorce proceedings. Within a few sessions John realizes that Barbara has made it clear, through body posturing and her liberal use of perfume, that she is attracted to him. The attraction is mutual, and John decides to engage in a consensual relationship with his patient.

What are the ethical implications of such a decision? What does the APTA Code of Ethics have to say about this? Discuss the ethical dilemma from a situational ethics standpoint, as well as from a classic ethical, principle-based perspective. What are the legal implications? Discuss practical approaches and solutions to this problem.

NOTE: The reader is encouraged to engage in a problem-solving exercise in which the same scenario is described but with John as the manager and Barbara as the staff physical therapist. How would this modification affect your analysis of the situation?

EMPLOYMENT LAW CONSIDERATIONS

Physical therapist managers are constantly dealing with issues involving employment law. Those individuals who function without the guidance of a human resource management department must deal with contracts, hiring and firing, performance appraisals, employee benefits, and regulatory schemes controlled by federal and state law. This section reviews basic employment law and introduces selected federal laws and agencies.

Employment at Will

Employment at will is a very old common law concept that simply means employers have a right to terminate their employees at any time, without advance notice, for any reason not contrary to law. In other words, they may terminate for good cause, bad cause, or no cause at all. Similarly, the employee is always free to resign from employment at any time. In theory, this structure creates a system in which neither party has an advantage. In employment at will situations, the employee is not under contract—there are no agreed-upon specific terms or duration. Most jurisdictions have laws such as these in place. However, there are many recognized exceptions to employment at will that have steadily eroded the doctrine; these exceptions represent an effort to afford employees greater protection from the unjustified acts of their employers.

Two of the generally recognized exceptions to employment at will are collective bargaining agreements and contracts for term. Since the 1920s, unions have been allowed to collectively bargain for their members. Union contracts provide security for their members who may be fired but not without a showing of just cause and not before participating in a union-approved grievance procedure. Contracts for term are something of a quasi-exception. Anyone who has a contract for term (e.g., a 2-year contract) may still be terminated but would have to be paid for the amount remaining on the contract.

Additional exceptions have evolved from public policy decisions to protect certain types of employee conduct. Employees terminated for conduct that society encourages may file **wrongful termination** lawsuits. Examples of public policy exceptions to employment at will include employees terminated for consulting with an attorney or serving on a jury. Another exception protects so-called whistleblowers, employees who are fired because they made a good faith report of a suspected violation of law to the authorities. If the federal government is the party being defrauded, the employee/plaintiff can file a **Qui tam** lawsuit under the False Claims Act (31 U.S.C. § 3729). *Qui tam*, a civil action (there are only monetary penalties), is loosely translated as "he who brings an action for the king as well as for himself." The original False Claims Act was signed into law by President Abraham Lincoln in 1863 to punish profiteers who sold the Union army shoddy supplies at inflated prices during the Civil War. Under the current False Claims Act, violators are liable for three times the dollar amount that the government is defrauded (i.e., treble damages). The person bringing the lawsuit may be able to share between 15% and 30% of the total recovery. In addition, the plaintiff may be entitled to reinstatement, double back pay, and special damages. The False Claims Act also protects the employee from demotion, harassment, or discrimination. It does not cover tax fraud or general waste and mismanagement.

As noted previously, contracts serve as a quasi-exception to the employment at will doctrine, in that they afford the employee additional protections against termination. Physical therapist employers and managers are urged to carefully review their employee handbooks. The legal literature is fraught with cases involving employees' claims that their handbooks constituted an employment contract. Ambiguities are generally decided in favor of the employee and might transform the at-will employment to an employment terminable only upon a finding of just cause. For example, if an employee handbook contained a clause indicating that "any and all disputes arising out of employment with the company will be resolved through arbitration," the company would generally be bound by that clause, even in the absence of an individual employment contract.

Employers and managers are also cautioned against making specific promises to employees that they do not intend to keep. If, for example, an employee was promised a transfer to a different city and moved his family, only to be terminated within 3 weeks of the move, he might be able to successfully sue for wrongful termination under the legal theory of Promissory Estoppel. The common law elements of promissory estoppel are as follows: (1) There must be a clear promise; (2) the employee relied on that promise; (3) the reliance was reasonable and foreseeable; and (4) the party claiming the reliance must have been injured by the promise. Courts view these types of scenarios as implied contracts between the employer and employee.

Additional public policy exceptions to the employment at will doctrine are based on state and federal constitutions, legislation, and administrative rules and regulations.

Employers cannot terminate employees in violation of The Civil Rights Acts, The Americans with Disability Act, The Age Discrimination in Employment Act, or other federal schemes that are discussed in more detail later in this chapter.

Employee Versus Independent Contractor

The distinction between employee and independent contractor carries with it significant consequences for both parties. The independent contractor, by definition, works outside of the control of the employer. When the question of whether someone is an independent contractor or an employee is raised, it is often in the context of tax liability. Therefore many of the distinguishing factors between the two are discussed in the Internal Revenue Service's (IRS's) regulations. **Independent contractors** must pay their own taxes and their own malpractice, disability, and worker's compensation premiums. They are not allowed to draw unemployment benefits. The key factor in distinguishing between employee and independent contractor lies in the control that the employer exerts over the actions of the individual. The more control exerted, the more likely it is that the court (or an agency such as the IRS) would classify the individual as an employee. In the physical therapy setting, control issues might include scheduling, patient flow, who is responsible for performance, who pays for liability insurance, and who pays for benefits. Courts view the "right to control" an individual's actions the same as "actual control."

Once this distinction is made, the employer is generally not liable for the acts of the independent contractor. However, the employer will still be primarily liable for the negligent selection and retention of independent contractors and for the failure to monitor the quality of care delivered within the organization, regardless of who delivers the care. Employers may also be liable for the conduct of contractors, under the theory of apparent agency, when they cannot be distinguished from employees in the eyes of the public.

Employment-Related Torts

Employment-related torts are civil suits, generally brought along with claims of wrongful termination. They may occur as a result of improperly conducted workplace investigations.

Defamation

Defamation is a false publication that injures a person's reputation in the community. These claims may be based on slander, when the defamatory communication is transmitted (published) orally, or libel, when the defamatory communication is transmitted by writing, video, or any other such mechanisms. An individual may defame another person or a business. The defamation may be per se, in which the communication is overtly injurious, or per quod, in which the injury is implied. In other words, per quod defamation applies if any reasonable person would assume that the communication was injurious to the reputation of the person or business. If the defamation is per se, then the plaintiff will most often prevail.

When someone alleges that he or she has been defamed, several defenses may be offered. Truth is always the best defense and usually ends the action. When the defendant can prove by a preponderance of the evidence that what he or she communicated was, in fact, the truth, the plaintiff will not prevail. Public policy has created additional defenses to claims of defamation. Qualified privilege generally attaches to criticism of official conduct (e.g., public employees, government officials, political appointees). As long as the person making the statement about these individuals can show that he or she acted in good faith, without actual knowledge of the falsity of the information, and did not offer the information in reckless disregard of the truth, the defendant will not be liable for defamation. The seminal case on this issue is *New York Times v. Sullivan*.[23] In that case, the U.S. Supreme Court set forth a standard that "prohibits a public official from recovering damages for a defamatory falsehood relating to his official conduct unless he proves that the statement was made with 'actual malice'—that is, with knowledge that it was false or with reckless disregard of whether it was false or not."

Under a variety of reporting statutes, physical therapists and other health care providers enjoy a qualified privilege against claims of defamation. For example, if a physical therapist suspected that a pediatric patient was a victim of child abuse and (in good faith) reported the parents to the proper authorities, the parents would not be able to bring a defamation claim against the therapist. In addition, physical therapists may enjoy qualified immunity when functioning in their official capacity as members of a government-appointed board, such as a State License Board. If the Board were to allege that a licensee violated the Code of Ethics or the state practice act, the respondent would generally not be allowed to claim that the board had defamed him.

Public policy has also dictated that in some states, expressions of opinions by members of the media (their own opinions, not the reported opinions of others) enjoy absolute privilege. Whereas qualified privilege can be defeated by a showing that there was knowledge of the falsity of the statement or malice, an absolute privilege cannot be defeated. Sitting judges and elected officials acting in their official capacity are thought to enjoy absolute privilege.

Negligent Hiring

Another employment-related tort is **negligent hiring**. In a Massachusetts case, *Ward v. Trusted Health*,[49] a supervisor at a program run by the Visiting Nurses Association (VNA) of Boston hired a home health aide with a criminal record.[49] Neither the program nor the VNA ran a background check on the aide, which would have shown six larceny-related convictions and the fact that the aide lied about his educational and work history on his application. The aide beat and stabbed to death the quadriplegic patient in his care in an attempt to cover up his thefts from the household. The patient's estate sued the home health agency and the VNA for negligent hiring and was awarded $26.5 million in damages.

Risk Management: Avoid Negligent Hiring

- Obtain a written consent to check references.
- Document all inquiries.
- Require applicant to certify that all information is true.
- Have applicant consent to credit check.
- Ask for copy of professional license, and contact license board to ensure its authenticity.

Letters of Recommendation

Physical therapist managers and supervisory personnel should also exercise caution when writing letters of recommendation. The practice of most Fortune 500 companies is to provide a letter that confirms dates of employment, salary, and little else. The risk of a defamation lawsuit precludes providing additional information. In an interesting case, an employee resigned (most likely under duress) and signed a settlement agreement stating that the employer would volunteer only the dates of employment, rate of pay, positions held, and so forth if queried by a potential new employer.[19] The former employer then proceeded to tell a prospective employer why the employee was fired and why he would not be rehired. The former employee subsequently sued for defamation and breach of contract. Because truth is a complete defense to defamation, the former employer prevailed on the defamation claim but was nonetheless found liable for breach of contract.

False-positive **references** might also pose potential problems. Employers could find themselves liable for positive statements in a letter of recommendation if either of the following applies: (1) The statements amount to affirmative misrepresentations or misleading half truths; or (2) the former employer knows that there is a foreseeable and substantial risk of physical harm to a prospective employer or third party. In a case on point, a school district provided a positive reference for a teacher who was a known child molester.[31] The teacher went on to molest a student in the new district, and the victim's parents successfully sued the former employer for providing a false-positive reference.

Invasion of Privacy and Intentional Infliction of Emotional Distress

Finally, employers and managers should be aware of the possibility of claims of invasion of privacy or intentional infliction of emotional distress. Both of these claims, especially the latter, carry significant difficulty in meeting the burden of proof. Invasion of privacy might involve a therapist's public disclosure of facts private to a patient (or employee), such as human immunovirus (HIV) status, sexual orientation, alcoholism, and drug use. Employers are cautioned to remember that when it comes to searching through the employee's area, the legitimate needs of the business are balanced against the employee's reasonable expectation of privacy. Personal belongings, lockers assigned to the employee, and desk drawers to which the employee has been issued a key should not be violated without a good excuse. The employee handbook should be very clear as to what the employer and employee should expect.

Plaintiff/employees can claim intentional infliction of emotional distress when the conduct of the employer or their agent so exceeds the bounds of decency that it would be considered atrocious and intolerable in a civilized community. Such extreme and outrageous conduct would be expected to cause severe emotional disturbances. Proving such a claim requires expert testimony to support the severe physical and psychological injury that the plaintiff will have to demonstrate he or she suffered as a result of the employer's conduct. Courts generally consider such conduct in context, recognizing that there are some very emotional situations in which a person might be expected to endure the resultant antagonism and mental anguish.

The Covenant Not to Compete in Employment Contracts

Although a full discussion of contract issues is beyond the scope of this chapter, a review of restrictive covenants (noncompete clauses) is worthwhile. Restrictive covenants place limitations on the parties to a contract. The covenant not to compete is a promise that the employee makes with his current or former employer. Courts generally do not favor such covenants because of the public policy argument against restraint of trade. However, when these covenants are tailored so as to promote the legitimate business interests of the employer while at the same time allowing the employee to work, the courts will enforce them. It is important to note that when and if these issues are raised in the courts, each case represents a unique set of facts within a particular employment setting. Therefore it is difficult to generalize as to which covenants will be enforced and which will not. Covenants not to compete, when enforced, must be reasonable in geographic scope and time. Most courts will enforce clauses that are 1 to 2 years in duration. Some courts will enforce these covenants only when the time employed exceeds the length of the covenant duration. The geographic scope varies according to the region. Generally, the more populated the region, the smaller the area-of-practice restriction. Courts tend to favor professional mobility and access to care. Therefore the courts may, on occasion, consider the direct impact of a restrictive covenant on patient care. For example, if a physical therapist signed a noncompete clause with a home health agency in a very rural area, the courts might decide that the contract was unreasonable (regardless of the duration or geographic scope) if it could be shown that by denying the therapist the ability to work, patients would not be served. With physician contracts, the courts may, in the interests of public policy, choose not to uphold such contracts if it can be shown that the physician-patient relationship would be adversely affected.

In addition to duration and geographic scope, the courts will look at specific practice restrictions and consideration. Covenants not to compete have the greatest chance of being upheld when they are narrowly tailored. For example, a covenant restricting the ability of a physical therapist who is Board-certified in pediatrics to open a private practice devoted to treating children within 1 mile of her former pediatric practice could not be used to restrict the same therapist from working as a generalist in the hospital across the street. With such an example, one can begin to see how the legitimate business interests of the former employer are balanced against the ability of the employee to earn a living.

To be valid and enforceable, the covenant not to compete must also be supported by consideration—that is, there must have been a bargained-for exchange and the employee must receive some form of value in exchange for the promise not to compete. The concept of consideration is a fundamental principle of contract law. Some courts have held that restrictive covenants are often the result of unequal bargaining power and thus need to be supported by new considerations, such as a raise or promotion. Other courts have allowed continued employment to serve as adequate consideration.

CASE STUDY 4-3

John is a physical therapist applying for the position of staff physical therapist. He has 2 years of experience and graduated from a well-respected program with an entry-level master's degree. His past 2 years of employment were spent at a large university-based medical center rotating through inpatient and outpatient duties on the orthopedic team. He has plans to sit for his board certification in orthopedics (OCS) within the next year. John is moving to state XYZ, where Gina's practice is located in the town of Zeena. He has already applied for, and received, licensure in XYZ.

Gina owns a moderately sized (three physical therapists, one physical therapist assistant, and a full-time aide) physical therapy practice in Zeena (population 50,000). She has been in business for 15 years and has a solid reputation. At least 80% of her referrals come from family practice physicians. Gina's practice is heavily weighted toward Medicare patients (Zeena is a retirement community), and she is boarded in geriatrics (GCS). She is looking to replace one of the physical therapists in her practice who recently moved out of town.

Gina's practice did well last year. Her overhead is low, and she can afford to offer a reasonable salary. The two remaining staff physical therapists have been with her practice for 5 years, and each earns approximately $50,000 per year. However, if she brings John on board, she would want assurance that he won't leave her practice to go work for the only other such business in town: the local hospital. The hospital is fully staffed, although it has a rather bad reputation and turnover is usually quite high.

The town is in a rural part of the state, and John would have to travel 50 miles each way for any other position in physical therapy. Gina wants John to sign the following noncompete clause:

The Employee recognizes that, due to the highly competitive businesses in which the Employer is engaged, personal contact is of primary importance in securing new patients/clients, retaining the goodwill of present patients/clients, and protecting the business of Employer. The Employee therefore agrees that during the time he is employed

CASE STUDY 4-3

by Employer and for a period of two (2) years after the termination of Employee's employment, he will not, within twenty-five (25) miles of the City of Zeena as an owner, officer, director, stockholder, tender, investor, principal, agent, partner, employee, consultant, distributor, dealer, contractor, broker, or trustee of any corporation, partnership, limited liability company, association, agency, proprietorship, joint venture, or any other entity of any nature, engage directly or indirectly, in any business of physical therapy that competes with Employer.

The Employee further agrees that for a period of two (2) years after the termination of Employee's employment, neither he nor any other person or business entity with which he may be affiliated in any capacity, will directly or indirectly (i) induce any patients/clients of the Employer to patronize any similar business which competes with the Employer; (ii) canvass, solicit, or accept any similar business from any patient/client of the Employer; (iii) directly or indirectly request or advise any patient/clients of the Employer to withdraw, curtail, or cancel such patient/client's business with the Employer; (iv) solicit or induce any employee of Employer to work for or with a business which competes with the Employer; or (v) directly or indirectly disclose to any other person, firm or corporation the names or addresses of any of the patient/clients of the Employer.

The period of time set forth above will be extended for a period of time equal to the time any litigation instituted by the employer to enforce the provisions herein remains pending.

If the provisions of this agreement are violated, in whole or in part, the Employer will be entitled, upon application to any court of proper jurisdiction, to a temporary restraining order or preliminary injunction to restrain and enjoin the Employee from such violation without prejudice to any other remedies the Employer may have at law or in equity. If the Employee violates this agreement, the Employee agrees that it would be impossible for the Employer to calculate its monetary damages and that the Employer would be irreparably harmed.

In the event that the provisions of this agreement are deemed to exceed the time, geographic, or occupational limitations permitted under applicable laws, the Employee and the Employer intend that any court with competent jurisdiction reform this agreement to provide for the maximum time, geographic, or occupational limitations permitted by applicable law.

DISCUSSION OF CASE STUDY 4-3

This particular covenant is vague and overly broad. Although Zeena is fairly rural, 25 miles is an unacceptable geographic scope, and John should consider reducing the duration to 1-year post employment. The clause is not tailored to a specific practice area, and there is no evidence of sufficient consideration beyond the employment contract itself. In addition, a fair reading of the contract would mean that John could not treat any former patient, for any reason, if he went to work at the hospital. The restrictive covenant is too heavily weighted in favor of the employer, and it is doubtful that the courts would enforce it.

This example of a noncompete clause was taken from an actual contract I reviewed for a physician. Although legalistic and wordy, its language is fairly standard. John should have his contract reviewed by a lawyer licensed to practice in State XYZ. He and his lawyer may opt to rewrite the clause in plainer language.

INTRODUCTION TO SELECTED FEDERAL LAWS AND AGENCIES

The following represents an overview of federal law that specifically addresses employment discrimination. In addition, the **Family Medical Leave Act** (FMLA) is reviewed.

Several federal laws prohibit job discrimination, among them Title VII of the **Civil Rights Act of 1964**,[6,7] **The Civil Rights Act of 1991**,[8] the Age Discrimination in Employment Act of 1967 (ADEA), and **Title I of the Americans with Disabilities Act of 1990** (ADA). The Equal Opportunities Commission (EEOC) enforces all of these laws. The EEOC promulgates rules and regulations and coordinates all federal actions related to employment practices. Owners of physical therapy practices, managers, and supervisors (especially those involved in hiring, firing, and the application of benefits) should be aware of the federal laws that control their actions and should take the time to review the EEOC's rules and regulations.

Civil Rights Act of 1964, Title VII

Congress enacted the Civil Rights Act in 1964 to remedy the discrimination and injustices suffered by minorities. The Act prohibits employment discrimination based on race, ethnicity, religion, and national origin. In 1972, gender was added to the roster of groups that have historically faced discrimination. These groups of individuals have come to be known as *protected classes*. Title VII applies to all private sector businesses with 15 or more employees; labor unions; and federal, state, and local governments. The Act prohibits both intentional and unintentional discrimination throughout the entire employment process (i.e., against job applicants as well as employees). Title VII, as with the ADA and ADEA, makes it illegal to discriminate in any aspect of employment, including hiring and firing, compensation, transfers, promotion, recruitment, testing; and training programs. Title VII is also the legal basis for sexual harassment claims in the workplace. Discriminatory practices under these laws include harassment; retaliation against an employee for alleging discrimination; employment decisions based on stereotypical assumptions; and denial of employment opportunities because of race, sex, religion, or association with a protected class.

There are a few circumstances in which overt discrimination is acceptable, such as when a bona fide occupational qualification (BFOQ) exists. For example, it would be acceptable to interview or hire only female applicants for the position of dressing room attendant in a woman's clothing store. Similarly, a Catholic church may choose to hire only Catholics—especially for clergy positions. However, employers should tread lightly when they decide to discriminate in any aspect of their employment process.

The Civil Rights Act of 1991

In 1991, Congress enacted legislation to amend the Civil Rights Act of 1964 in an effort to "strengthen and improve federal civil rights laws, to provide for damages in cases of intentional employment discrimination, to clarify provisions regarding disparate impact actions, and for other purposes."[8] The Civil Rights Act of 1991 was specifically enacted to provide "additional remedies under federal law ... to deter unlawful harassment and intentional discrimination in the workplace; [and to] provide additional protections against unlawful discrimination in employment." The Act reversed several Supreme Court decisions that limited the rights of persons protected by these laws. It provides for obtaining attorneys' fees and the possibility of jury trials. It also directs the EEOC to expand its technical assistance and outreach activities.

The Age Discrimination in Employment Act of 1973

The **Age Discrimination in Employment Act (ADEA)** prohibits employers from discriminating on the basis of age.[40] This applies to private companies with 20 or more employees, including state and local governments. It also applies to employment agencies, labor organizations, and the federal government.

The prohibited practices are nearly identical to those outlined in Title VII because many provisions of the ADEA were modeled on the Civil Rights Act. An employee is protected from discrimination on the basis of age if he or she is over 40. It was previously held that if an employee was terminated and replaced with an individual over the age of 40, then he or she would not be able to sue on the basis of age discrimination. However, in *O'Conner v. Consolidated Coin Caterers Corp.*, the U.S. Supreme Court held that a plaintiff is required to show only that he or she was replaced by a "substantially younger" individual.[25] It is also unlawful to retaliate against an employee for opposing practices that violate the Act or for filing a claim or testifying in an ADEA case. As with Title VII, it is permissible for an employer to specify age limits in rare circumstances in which age has been proven to be a bona fide occupational qualification.

In a more recent United States Supreme Court case (*General Dynamics Land Systems Inc. v. Cline et al*),[15] a collective bargaining agreement eliminated the company's obligation to provide health benefits to subsequently retired employees, except as to then-current workers who were 50 years of age or older. The employees who were then at least 40 (covered by ADEA) but under 50 years old claimed that the agreement violated the ADEA, constituting a type of reverse age discrimination. The Supreme Court held that the ADEA's text, structure, purpose, history, and relationship to other federal statutes combined to show that the statute was not intended to stop an employer from favoring an older employee over a younger one, even though both were covered under the law. Thus the plaintiffs-employees, all between 40 and 50 years old, who were denied health benefits under the terms of a collective bargaining agreement were not protected by ADEA.

The ADEA contains no explicit prohibition against asking a prospective employee's age or date of birth. However, employers should realize that because such questions may deter older individuals from applying or may appear to be discriminatory, they will be closely scrutinized to ensure that the question was made for a lawful purpose.

The ADEA's ban against age discrimination also prohibits denial of benefits to older employees. An employer may reduce benefits on the basis of age only if the cost of providing the reduced benefits to older workers is the same as the cost of providing benefits to younger workers. Under ADEA, an individual may agree to waive his rights at the employer's request. This might occur, for example, during a "rightsizing" of the company. However, the waiver must be knowing and voluntary (completely understood and freely given) in order to be valid. Among other requirements, a valid ADEA waiver must conform to the following: (1) It must be in writing and be understandable; (2) it must specifically refer to ADEA rights or claims; (3) it may not waive rights or claims that may arise in the future; (4) it must be in exchange for valuable consideration; (5) it must advise the individual in writing to seek an attorney before signing the waiver; and (6) it must provide the individual at least 21 days to consider the agreement and at least 7 days to revoke.

The Americans With Disabilities Act of 1990

On July 26, 1990, President George H.W. Bush signed into law The Americans with Disabilities Act (ADA). This piece of civil rights legislation prohibits employment discrimination against qualified individuals with disabilities. The ADA currently applies to private employers, state and local governments, employment agencies, labor unions, and joint labor-management committees that employ 15 or more individuals. The ADA covers all aspects of the employment process (e.g., application, testing, hiring, promotion, medical examinations). To ensure nondiscrimination, the ADA requires employers to make **reasonable accommodations** for the qualified applicant or employee with a disability, unless it can be shown that the accommodation would cause an **undue hardship** for the employer.

The legislative precursor of the ADA was The Rehabilitation Act of 1973. The Rehabilitation Act referred to "handicaps" rather than *disabilities*. The Rehabilitation Act applies only to the federal government, federal contractors, and agencies receiving federal funds. As such, it is more narrowly applied than the ADA, which, in contrast, affects the private sector. Any disabled individual can file a claim under the ADA, regardless of his or her employer. Unlike the ADA, The Rehabilitation Act's regulations do not define **essential function** (discussed in more detail later).

In passing the ADA, Congress has noted that individuals with disabilities are a "discrete and insular minority with a history of being subjected to discrimination."[41] Before implementation of the ADA, these individuals did not always have an available mechanism to redress discrimination. By enacting the ADA, Congress sought to "provide a clear and comprehensive national mandate for the elimination of discrimination against individuals with disabilities." The EEOC is charged with enforcing the ADA. The regulations to implement the equal employment provisions (Title I) of the ADA are found in 29 C.F.R. § 1630 (1991).[47] The EEOC also provides an appendix to part 1630—Interpretive Guidance on Title I of the ADA.

The ADA is divided into five titles:
- Title I deals with employment discrimination and calls for reasonable accommodations to protect the rights of disabled persons.
- Title II requires that public services (e.g., public transportation) are accessible.
- Title III relates to public accommodations and mandates that all new construction be accessible to individuals with disabilities.
- Title IV requires accommodations to be made within the telecommunications industry, especially for the deaf.
- Title V is a miscellaneous provision that, among other things, prohibits threats and retaliation against disabled persons.

Disability

The purpose of Title I of the ADA is to ensure that qualified individuals with disabilities are not discriminated against because of their disability. With respect to an individual, the ADA broadly defines disability as follows: (1) a physical or mental impairment that substantially limits one or more of that person's major life activities; (2) having a record of such an impairment; and (3) being regarded as having such an impairment. To qualify as disabled under the ADA, an individual must meet one of these three requirements. Physical impairments include physiological disorders or conditions affecting the various body systems (e.g., neurological, musculoskeletal, special sense organs). However, the ADA does not supply an exhaustive list of impairments. Rather, the disability is determined by the effect of the impairment on the life of the individual. The impairment must substantially limit a major life activity. *Major life activities* are defined as functions such as caring for oneself, hearing, seeing, walking, and breathing. A major life activity is a basic activity performed by the average person in the general population with little or no difficulty. An impairment substantially limits a major life activity if, because of that impairment, the individual is unable to perform that major life activity. The impairment is also said to substantially limit a major life activity if there is a significant restriction in the condition, manner, or duration under which an individual can perform a major life activity. For example, an individual who, because of his or her impairment, could sit only for brief periods of time would be limited in the major life activity of sitting. Such an individual would be significantly restricted in the ability to perform a broad range of jobs compared with the average person having comparable training. The ADA supplies factors to be considered in determining whether an individual is substantially limited in a major life activity.

Having a record of impairment means that an individual with a history of a qualified impairment is still considered disabled. For example, an alcoholic who was not drinking would still be protected from discrimination on the basis of his or her prior medical history. The third requirement of a disability is being regarded as having such an impairment. Even in the absence of an impairment that does not substantially limit a major life activity, individuals may be regarded as having such an impairment if they are perceived by a covered entity (e.g., employers) as having such a limitation.

The ADA prohibits discrimination on the basis of disability against qualified individuals with disabilities. The ADA defines a qualified individual with a disability as "an individual with a disability who satisfies the requisite skill, experience, education, and other job-related requirements of the employment position such individual holds or desires, and who, with or without reasonable accommodation, can perform the essential functions of such position." Thus a two-step process is employed to determine if an individual is qualified. First, the individual must possess the appropriate education, licensure, employment experience, and so forth. For example, an applicant for a position as a physical therapist must first possess a license to practice as a physical therapist regardless of any disability. Second, the individual must be able to perform the essential functions of the position, with or without reasonable accommodation.

Essential Functions

The essential functions are the fundamental job duties of the employment position. The term *essential functions* does not include the marginal (nonessential) functions of the position. The individual who holds a position must be able to perform essential functions either unaided or with reasonable accommodation.

Various factors are applied to determine whether a particular function is essential to that position. If a position exists only to perform a particular function, the function is essential. For example, if a person is hired to be a typist, the ability to type would be an essential function. A second factor is if there are a limited number of employees among whom the job can be distributed. If an employer has a small number of employees, each employee may have to perform several tasks and each position therefore will have multiple essential functions. A third factor is if the function is highly specialized and if the person in that position is hired for his or her expertise. Other factors may be considered, such as the consequences of failing to require the employee to perform the function. For example, although the ability to hear is only one function of a physical therapist, being unable to hear at all must be considered when determining the essential functions of that position.

The aforementioned list of factors is not exhaustive. Whether a function is essential is to be determined on a case-by-case basis. If the employer asserts that a function is essential, the employee must be required actually to perform that function. For example, lifting patients may be listed in the job description of an employee hired as a physical therapist, but the employer who owns a practice devoted to hand therapy may not ever need an employee to lift a patient. Therefore lifting patients is not actually an essential function of that position. In contrast, if a job description lists manual therapy as only one aspect of a physical therapy position but the employee spends most of his or her time doing manual techniques, then manual therapy would be an essential function.

Reasonable Accommodation

An accommodation is a "change in the work environment or in the way things are customarily done that enables an individual with a disability to enjoy equal employment opportunities."[47] Accommodations can be made in the application process, in the job itself, or to enable the enjoyment of equal benefits and privileges by employees with disabilities. The EEOC regulations provide several examples of reasonable accommodation. An employer may make a reasonable accommodation by making the physical facilities readily accessible or by job restructuring. Job restructuring may be accomplished by reallocating marginal job functions to a nondisabled employee.

The Office of Disability Employment Policy of the U.S. Department of Labor supports the Job Accommodation Network (JAN), a free consulting service designed to increase the employability of people with disabilities. This web site, located at http://www.jan.wvu.edu/, provides individualized worksite accommodation solutions and technical assistance regarding the ADA and other disability-related legislation.

Undue Hardship

The ADA provides for defenses to charges of discrimination. With respect to reasonable accommodation, the defense of undue hardship may be available. *Undue hardship* means that the employer would incur significant expense in an attempt to accommodate. Several factors are to be considered in determining whether undue hardship exists. Among these factors are the nature and cost of the accommodation, the overall financial resources of the employer, the number of employees, and the impact of the accommodation on the operation of the facility. Even if the employer can show an undue hardship, accommodation may still be required if the funding is available from another source (e.g., state or federal agencies). Also, undue hardship is not limited to financial considerations. It could refer to any accommodation that would have a disruptive effect on a business, its customers, or other employees. For example, if dim lighting is part of the atmosphere of a nightclub, the nightclub would not be required to change the lighting (an inexpensive accommodation) for the benefit of a visually impaired waiter, even if that individual would be able to perform the job in bright lighting.

Determining Essential Functions

Good job descriptions identify the essential job functions. Good job descriptions are not overly inclusive and do not state irrelevant information. However, the employer should aim for flexibility by stating that the position is subject to the assignment of new duties. Employers would be wise to observe and interview those currently performing a particular job before creating both the job description and the essential job functions. Printed job descriptions have a presumption of credibility if they were published before the job posting or interview.

EMPLOYER CONSIDERATIONS IN HIRING

Under the ADA, the employer is not permitted to ask an applicant whether he or she is disabled or about the nature or severity of a disability; nor may an employer require the applicant to take a medical examination before making a job offer. However, the employer is permitted to ask questions about the applicant's ability to perform job-related functions as long as those questions are not phrased in terms of a disability. The employer may also ask an applicant to describe or demonstrate how, with or without reasonable accommodation, the applicant will perform job-related functions.

After an offer of employment is made, and before actual job duties commence, the applicant may be required to take a medical examination. The employer may condition the offer of employment on the results of the medical examination. However, employers are cautioned to remember that all potential employees (in that category or job classification) must be subjected to the same examination. If an individual is not hired because a medical examination reveals the existence of a disability, the employer still has the burden of demonstrating that the reasons for exclusion are related to business necessity. The results of all medical examinations or information about a disability must be kept confidential and maintained in separate medical files. Employers and managers are cautioned to refrain from writing any comments on a job application or résumé and to make all efforts to ensure that the interview and hiring process is the same for all candidates across the board.

It is also worth noting that although alcoholism and drug addiction may qualify as a disability, current illegal substance abusers are not protected by the ADA and may be denied employment or fired on the basis of such use. The ADA does not prevent employers from testing applicants or employees for current illegal drug use or from making employment decisions on the basis of verifiable results. A test for the illegal use of drugs is not considered a medical examination under the ADA; therefore it is not a prohibited pre-employment medical examination.

Recent U.S. Supreme Court Cases

In recent terms, the U.S. Supreme Court has decided several other cases, which significantly affect the interpretation of the ADA. In *Bragdon v. Abbott*,[4] the Supreme Court broadly interpreted the terms *impairment, major life activity,* and *substantial limitation,* holding that a woman with asymptomatic HIV infection had an ADA disability. In light of this case, the EEOC was instructed to continue to give a broad interpretation to these terms.

In 1999, the Supreme Court heard three cases related to the ADA. In *Sutton v. United Air Lines, Inc.*,[39] and *Murphy v. United Parcel Service, Inc.*,[21] the Court held that the determination of whether a person has an ADA-defined disability must take into consideration whether the person is substantially limited in a major life activity when using a mitigating measure, such as medication, a prosthesis, or a hearing aid. A person who experiences no substantial limitation in any major life activity when using a mitigating measure does not meet the ADA's first definition of *disability* (i.e., a physical or mental impairment that substantially limits a major life activity). In *Albertsons, Inc. v. Kirkingburg*,[1] the Court extended this analysis to individuals who specifically develop compensating behaviors to mitigate the effects of impairment. This ruling was in opposition to the EEOC's former position that the beneficial effects of mitigating measures should not be considered when determining whether a person meets the first definition of disability.

In the past 10 years, plaintiffs have filed an increasing number of ADA claims stating that they had an impairment that prevented them from performing a specific job function in the workplace and hence claiming they had a **qualified disability**. In *Toyota Motor Manufacturing v. Williams*,[45] the U.S. Supreme Court answered the following question: "Does a person who is limited in some, but not all, job-related tasks meet the definition of a disability?" In this landmark case, the Court stated that an individual must have an impairment that prevents or severely restricts activities that are of central importance to most people's daily lives rather than just to a particular job.

In all of these cases, the Supreme Court emphasized that the determination of whether a person has a disability must be made on a case-by-case basis. The Court has stated that it could not be assumed that everyone with a particular type of impairment who uses a particular mitigating measure automatically was included (or excluded) from the ADA's definition of disability.

The Family Medical Leave Act of 1993

The Family Medical Leave Act (FMLA), signed into law by President William Jefferson Clinton, is already proving to be one of the most significant pieces of employment legislation passed in the last decade. FMLA was designed to protect almost all workers, regardless of whether or not they belong to a protected class. FMLA allows for up to 12 weeks of unpaid job and benefit protection per year for serious personal and family health conditions. The employee is entitled to return to the same position or to an equivalent position with equivalent benefits, pay, status, and other terms and conditions of employment. The Act covers state, local, and federal employees; local education agencies (schools); and private sector employers who employ 50 or more employees for at least 20 weeks in the current or preceding calendar year. In order to be covered, individual employees must have worked for their employer for a total of at least 12 months and a minimum of 1250 hours during the previous 12 months. Covered employees work either where there are 50 people employed or within 75 miles of that location.

Under FMLA, a serious health condition is defined as an "illness, injury or impairment, or physical or mental condition involving either inpatient care or continuing treatment by a health care provider."[42] Covered conditions include hospital care as an inpatient, any absence of greater than 3 days requiring treatment, and any period of incapacity related to pregnancy. Treatment for chronic conditions (e.g., asthma, diabetes, epilepsy), permanent or long-term conditions requiring supervision (e.g., Alzheimer's disease or terminal diseases), and conditions that require multiple treatments and would incapacitate if left untreated (e.g., chemotherapy) are also covered. Eligible employees may request protected leave for their own serious health condition or to care for a son, daughter, spouse, or parent.

The FMLA is much more of an entitlement than a protection against discriminatory conduct. Employees are not required to accept light duty work or any type of accommodation. The employee must schedule foreseeable leave so as not to unduly disrupt the employer's operations. In addition, the employee must give a 30-day notice for non-emergency leave, and the employer may require a certificate of illness or a second opinion (or both).

REFERENCES AND READINGS

1. *Albertsons, Inc. v. Kirkingburg*, 527 U.S. 555 (1999).
2. APTA Commissioned Survey on Sexual Harassment.
3. *Barvee v. Finerty* 100 Ohio App.3d 466. 1995.
4. *Bragdon v. Abbott*, 524 U.S. 624 (1998).
5. Civil Rights Act of 1964, Title VII, 42 USC, § 703(a).
6. Civil Rights Act of 1964, Title VII, 42 U.S.C. § 703 (e).
7. Civil Rights Act of 1964, Title VII, 42 U.S.C. §§ 2000e – 2000e17.
8. Civil Rights Act of 1991, Public Law 102-166, 105 Stat. 071, 42 U.S.C. §§ 1981 and 2000e. 703 (e).
9. CNA Physical Therapy Claims Study, 2006. (Accessed at http://www.cna.com/cnaeportal/vcm_content/CNA/internet/Static%20File%20for%20Download/Risk%20Control/Medical%20Services/Physical_Therapy_Claims_Study.pdf.)
10. *Code of ethics: guide for professional conduct*, Alexandria, Va, 2000, American Physical Therapy Association.
11. DeMayo RA: Patient sexual behaviors and sexual harassment: a national survey of physical therapists, *Physical Therapy* 77(7):739-744, 1997.
12. *Ellerth v. Burlington Industries, Inc.*, 524 U.S. 742 (1998).
13. Emanual EJ, Dubler NN: Preserving the physician-patient relationship in the era of managed care, *JAMA* 273:44, 323-329, 1995.
14. *Farragher v. City of Boca Raton*, 524 U.S. 775, 1998 and *Burlington Industries, Inc. v. Ellerth*, Case No. 97-569 (U.S. Supreme Court, June 26, 1998).
15. *General Dynamics Land Systems, Inc. v. Cline*, 540 U.S. 581, 2004.
16. *Guide to physical therapy practice*, ed 2, Alexandria, Va, 2003, American Physical Therapy Association.
17. Hiepler MO, Dunn BC: Irreconcilable differences: why the doctor-patient relationship is disintegrating at the hands of health maintenance organizations and Wall Street, *Pepperdine Law Review* 25(3): 9-28, 1998.
18. Levitt SJ, Oneill RJ: A call for a functional multidisciplinary approach to intervention in cases of elder abuse, neglect, and exploitation: one legal clinic's experience, *The Elder Law Journal* 5(1): 204, 1997.
19. *Love v. Univ. Cincinnati Hosp.* 90 Ohio Misc.2d. 4. (1997).
20. *Madera v. Satellite Shelters*, Inc., 86 Ohio St. 3d 1202, 1999.
21. *Murphy v. United Parcel Service, Inc.*, 527 U.S. 516 (1999).
22. *Neade v. Portes*, No. 2-97-1099 2nd District, Ill., March 31, 1999.
23. *New York Times v. Sullivan*, 376 U.S. 254 (1964).
24. Nolan JR, Nolan-Haley JM: *Black's law dictionary*, ed 6, St. Paul, 1990, West Publishing.

25. *O'Conner v. Consolidated Coin Caterers Corp*, 000 U.S. U10195 (Decided April 1, 1996).

26. *Oncale v. Sundowner Offshore Services, Inc.*, No. 96-568 (U.S. Supreme Court, March 4, 1998).

27. *Pegram v. Herdrich*, 530 U.S. 211 (2000).

28. *Procedural Document on Disciplinary Action of the American Physical Therapy Association*, Alexandria, Va, March 1996, American Physical Therapy Association.

29. *PT Magazine* – Charlene Portee Open Letter to Membership.

30. Purtilo, RB, Cassel C: *Ethical dimensions in the health care professions*, Philadelphia, 1988, Saunders.

31. *Randi v. Muroc Joint Unified School District*, 929 P. 2d 582 (1997).

32. Rozovsky FA: *Consent to treatment: a practical guide*, ed 2, Boston, 1990, Little and Brown.

33. Salladay SA: Rehabilitation, ethics and managed care, *REHAB Management*, pp. 38-42, October/November 1996.

34. Scott RW: *Health care malpractice*, ed 2, New York, 1999, McGraw-Hill.

35. Scott RW: *Professional ethics: a guide for rehabilitation professionals*, St Louis, 1998, Mosby.

36. Scott RW: *Promoting legal awareness in physical and occupational therapy*, St Louis, 1997, Mosby.

37. Sex Discrimination Guidelines, Equal Employment Opportunity Commission, 29 CFR 1604.11, *Federal Register*, 45:74677, November 10, 1980.

38. *Standards of ethical conduct for the physical therapist assistant: guide for conduct of the affiliate member*, Alexandria, Va, 2000, American Physical Therapy Association.

39. *Sutton v. United Airlines, Inc.*, 527 U.S. 471, 67 U.S.L.W. 4537 (June 22, 1999).

40. The Age Discrimination in Employment Act of 1967, 29 USC. §§621-634.

41. The Americans with Disabilities Act of 1990, Pub.L.No. 101-336 (1990) found at 42 USC. §§12101 et seq.

42. The Family and Medical Leave Act of 1993, Public Law 103-3 (1993).

43. The Rehabilitation Act of 1973, 29 U.S.C. 790 et seq.

44. Title IX of the Educational Amendments of 1972, 42 USC, §§ 1681-1683.

45. *Toyota Motor Manufacturing v. Williams*, 534 U.S. 184, No. 00-1089 (2001).

46. Triezenberg HL: The identification of ethical issues in physical therapy practice, *Physical Therapy* 76(10):1097-1107, 1996.

47. 29 C.F.R. app. § 1630.2(o).

48. Velick MD: Mandatory reporting statutes: a necessary yet underutilized response to elder abuse, *The Elder Law Journal* 3:165, 1995. 24. Ohio Rev. Code § 3721.13 (A)(13).

49. *Ward v. Trusted Health*, No. 94-4297 (Suffolk Sup. Ct.).

49a. Weber DO: Who's sorry now, *Physician Executive* 32(2):6, 11-14, 2006.

50. *Wickline v. The State of California*, 192 Cal. App. 33d. 1630.1986.

51. Wynia MK, Latham SR, Kao AC: Medical professionalism in society, *New England Journal of Medicine* 341(21):1612-1616, 1999.

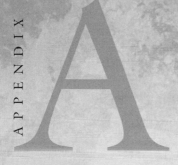

APPENDIX **A**

American Physical Therapy Association Code of Ethics and Guide for Professional Conduct

APTA Code of Ethics

HOD 06-00-12-23 (Program 17) [Amended HOD 06-91-05-05; HOD 06-87-11-17; HOD 06-81-06-18; HOD 06-78-06-08; HOD 06-78-06-07, HOD 06-77-18-30; HOD 06-77-17-27; Initial HOD 06-73-13-24]

Preamble
This Code of Ethics of the American Physical Therapy Association sets forth principles for the ethical practice of physical therapy. All physical therapists are responsible for maintaining and promoting ethical practice. To this end, the physical therapist shall act in the best interest of the patient/client. This Code of Ethics shall be binding on all physical therapists.

Principle 1
A physical therapist shall respect the rights and dignity of all individuals and shall provide compassionate care.

Principle 2
A physical therapist shall act in a trustworthy manner towards patients/clients and in all other aspects of physical therapy practice.

Principle 3
A physical therapist shall comply with laws and regulations governing physical therapy and shall strive to effect changes that benefit patients/clients.

Principle 4
A physical therapist shall exercise sound professional judgment.

Principle 5
A physical therapist shall achieve and maintain professional competence.

Principle 6
A physical therapist shall maintain and promote high standards for physical therapy practice, education, and research.

Principle 7
A physical therapist shall seek only such remuneration as is deserved and reasonable for physical therapy services.

Principle 8
A physical therapist shall provide and make available accurate and relevant information to patients/clients about their care and to the public about physical therapy services.

Principle 9
A physical therapist shall protect the public and the profession from unethical, incompetent, and illegal acts.

Principle 10
A physical therapist shall endeavor to address the health needs of society.

Principle 11
A physical therapist shall respect the rights, knowledge, and skills of colleagues and other health care professionals.

APTA Guide for Professional Conduct

Purpose
This Guide for Professional Conduct (Guide) is intended to serve physical therapists in interpreting the Code of Ethics (Code) of the American Physical Therapy Association (Association), in matters of professional conduct. The Guide provides guidelines by which physical therapists may determine the propriety of their conduct. It is also intended to guide the professional development of physical therapist students. The Code and the Guide apply to all physical therapists. These guidelines are subject to change as the dynamics of the profession change and as new patterns of health care delivery are developed and accepted by the professional community and the public. This Guide is subject to monitoring and timely revision by the Ethics and Judicial Committee of the Association.

Interpreting Ethical Principles
The interpretations expressed in this Guide reflect the opinions, decisions, and advice of the Ethics and Judicial Committee. These interpretations are intended to assist a physical therapist in applying general ethical principles to specific situations. They should not be considered inclusive of all situations that could evolve.

Principle 1

A physical therapist shall respect the rights and dignity of all individuals and shall provide compassionate care.

1.1 Attitudes of a Physical Therapist

A. A physical therapist shall recognize, respect, and respond to individual and cultural differences with compassion and sensitivity.
B. A physical therapist shall be guided at all times by concern for the physical, psychological, and socioeconomic welfare of patients/clients.
C. A physical therapist shall not harass, abuse, or discriminate against others.

Principle 2

A physical therapist shall act in a trustworthy manner toward patients/clients and in all other aspects of physical therapy practice.

2.1 Patient/Physical Therapist Relationship

A. A physical therapist shall place the patient/client's interest(s) above those of the physical therapist. Working in the patient/client's best interest requires knowledge of the patient/client's needs from the patient/client's perspective. Patients/clients often come to the physical therapist in a vulnerable state and normally will rely on the physical therapist's advice, which they perceive to be based on superior knowledge, skill, and experience. The trustworthy physical therapist acts to ameliorate the patient's/client's vulnerability, not to exploit it.
B. A physical therapist shall not exploit any aspect of the physical therapist/patient relationship.
C. A physical therapist shall not engage in any sexual relationship or activity, whether consensual or nonconsensual, with any patient while a physical therapist/patient relationship exists. Termination of the physical therapist/patient relationship does not eliminate the possibility that a sexual or intimate relationship may exploit the vulnerability of the former patient/client.
D. A physical therapist shall encourage an open and collaborative dialogue with the patient/client.
E. In the event the physical therapist or patient terminates the physical therapist/patient relationship while the patient continues to need physical therapy services, the physical therapist should take steps to transfer the care of the patient to another provider.

2.2 Truthfulness

A physical therapist has an obligation to provide accurate and truthful information. A physical therapist shall not make statements that he/she knows or should know are false, deceptive, fraudulent, or misleading. See Section 8.2.C and D.

2.3 Confidential Information

A. Information relating to the physical therapist/patient relationship is confidential and may not be communicated to a third party not involved in that patient's care without the prior consent of the patient, subject to applicable law.
B. Information derived from peer review shall be held confidential by the reviewer unless the physical therapist who was reviewed consents to the release of the information.
C. A physical therapist may disclose information to appropriate authorities when it is necessary to protect the welfare of an individual or the community or when required by law. Such disclosure shall be in accordance with applicable law.

2.4 Patient Autonomy and Consent

A. A physical therapist shall respect the patient's/client's right to make decisions regarding the recommended plan of care, including consent, modification, or refusal.
B. A physical therapist shall communicate to the patient/client the findings of his/her examination, evaluation, diagnosis, and prognosis.
C. A physical therapist shall collaborate with the patient/client to establish the goals of treatment and the plan of care.
D. A physical therapist shall use sound professional judgment in informing the patient/client of any substantial risks of the recommended examination and intervention.
E. A physical therapist shall not restrict patients' freedom to select their provider of physical therapy.

Principle 3

A physical therapist shall comply with laws and regulations governing physical therapy and shall strive to effect changes that benefit patients/clients.

3.1 Professional Practice

A physical therapist shall comply with laws governing the qualifications, functions, and duties of a physical therapist.

3.2 Just Laws and Regulations

A physical therapist shall advocate the adoption of laws, regulations, and policies by providers, employers, third-party payers, legislatures, and regulatory agencies to provide and improve access to necessary health care services for all individuals.

3.3 Unjust Laws and Regulations

A physical therapist shall endeavor to change unjust laws, regulations, and policies that govern the practice of physical therapy. See Section 10.2.

Principle 4

A physical therapist shall exercise sound professional judgment.

4.1 Professional Responsibility

A. A physical therapist shall make professional judgments that are in the patient/client's best interests.

B. Regardless of practice setting, a physical therapist has primary responsibility for the physical therapy care of a patient and shall make independent judgments regarding that care consistent with accepted professional standards. See Sections 2.4 and 6.1.

C. A physical therapist shall not provide physical therapy services to a patient/client while his/her ability to do so safely is impaired.

D. A physical therapist shall exercise sound professional judgment based upon his/her knowledge, skill, education, training, and experience.

E. Upon accepting a patient/client for physical therapy services, a physical therapist shall be responsible for the examination, evaluation, and diagnosis of that individual; the prognosis and intervention; re-examination and modification of the plan of care; and the maintenance of adequate records, including progress reports. A physical therapist shall establish the plan of care and shall provide and/or supervise and direct the appropriate interventions. See Section 2.4.

F. If the diagnostic process reveals findings that are outside the scope of the physical therapist's knowledge, experience, or expertise, the physical therapist shall so inform the patient/client and refer to an appropriate practitioner.

G. When the patient has been referred from another practitioner, the physical therapist shall communicate pertinent findings and/or information to the referring practitioner.

H. A physical therapist shall determine when a patient/client will no longer benefit from physical therapy services. See Section 7.1.D.

4.2 Direction and Supervision

A. The supervising physical therapist has primary responsibility for the physical therapy care rendered to a patient/client.

B. A physical therapist shall not delegate to a less qualified person any activity that requires the professional skill, knowledge, and judgment of the physical therapist.

4.3 Practice Arrangements

A. Participation in a business, partnership, corporation, or other entity does not exempt physical therapists, whether employers, partners, or stockholders, either individually or collectively, from the obligation to promote, maintain and comply with the ethical principles of the Association.

B. A physical therapist shall advise his/her employer(s) of any employer practice that causes a physical therapist to be in conflict with the ethical principles of the Association. A physical therapist shall seek to eliminate aspects of his/her employment that are in conflict with the ethical principles of the Association.

4.4 Gifts and Other Consideration(s)

A. A physical therapist shall not invite, accept, or offer gifts, monetary incentives, or other considerations that affect or give an appearance of affecting his/her professional judgment.

B. A physical therapist shall not offer or accept kickbacks in exchange for patient referrals. See Sections 7.1.F and G and 9.1.D.

Principle 5

A physical therapist shall achieve and maintain professional competence.

5.1 Scope of Competence

A physical therapist shall practice within the scope of his/her competence and commensurate with his/her level of education, training and experience.

5.2 Self-assessment

A physical therapist has a lifelong professional responsibility for maintaining competence through on-going self-assessment, education, and enhancement of knowledge and skills.

5.3 Professional Development

A physical therapist shall participate in educational activities that enhance his/her basic knowledge and skills. See Section 6.1.

Principle 6

A physical therapist shall maintain and promote high standards for physical therapy practice, education and research.

6.1 Professional Standards

A physical therapist's practice shall be consistent with accepted professional standards. A physical therapist shall continuously engage in assessment activities to determine compliance with these standards.

6.2 Practice

A. A physical therapist shall achieve and maintain professional competence. See Section 5.

B. A physical therapist shall demonstrate his/her commitment to quality improvement by engaging in peer and utilization review and other self-assessment activities.

6.3 Professional Education

A. A physical therapist shall support high-quality education in academic and clinical settings.

B. A physical therapist participating in the educational process is responsible to the students, the academic institutions, and the clinical settings for promoting ethical conduct. A physical therapist shall model ethical behavior and provide the student with information about the Code of Ethics, opportunities to discuss ethical conflicts, and procedures for reporting unresolved ethical conflicts. See Section 9.

6.4 Continuing Education

A. A physical therapist providing continuing education must be competent in the content area

B. When a physical therapist provides continuing education, he/she shall ensure that course content, objectives, faculty credentials, and responsibilities of the instructional staff are accurately stated in the promotional and instructional course materials.

C. A physical therapist shall evaluate the efficacy and effectiveness of information and techniques presented in continuing education programs before integrating them into his or her practice.

6.5 Research

A. A physical therapist participating in research shall abide by ethical standards governing protection of human subjects and dissemination of results.

B. A physical therapist shall support research activities that contribute knowledge for improved patient care.

C. A physical therapist shall report to appropriate authorities any acts in the conduct or presentation of research that appear unethical or illegal. See Section 9.

Principle 7

A physical therapist shall seek only such remuneration as is deserved and reasonable for physical therapy services.

7.1 Business and Employment Practices

A. A physical therapist's business/employment practices shall be consistent with the ethical principles of the Association.

B. A physical therapist shall never place her/his own financial interest above the welfare of individuals under his/her care.

C. A physical therapist shall recognize that third-party payer contracts may limit, in one form or another, the provision of physical therapy services. Third-party limitations do not absolve the physical therapist from making sound professional judgments that are in the patient's best interest. A physical therapist shall avoid underutilization of physical therapy services.

D. When a physical therapist's judgment is that a patient will receive negligible benefit from physical therapy services, the physical therapist shall not provide or continue to provide such services if the primary reason for doing so is to further the financial self-interest of the physical therapist or his/her employer. A physical therapist shall avoid overutilization of physical therapy services. See Section 4.1.H.

E. Fees for physical therapy services should be reasonable for the service performed, considering the setting in which it is provided, practice costs in the geographic area, judgment of other organizations, and other relevant factors.

F. A physical therapist shall not directly or indirectly request, receive, or participate in the dividing, transferring, assigning, or rebating of an unearned fee. See Sections 4.4.A and B.

G. A physical therapist shall not profit by means of a credit or other valuable consideration, such as an unearned commission, discount, or gratuity, in connection with the furnishing of physical therapy services. See Sections 4.4.A and B.

H. Unless laws impose restrictions to the contrary, physical therapists who provide physical therapy services within a business entity may pool fees and monies received. Physical therapists may divide or apportion these fees and monies in accordance with the business agreement.

I. A physical therapist may enter into agreements with organizations to provide physical therapy services if such agreements do not violate the ethical principles of the Association or applicable laws.

7.2 Endorsement of Products or Services

A. A physical therapist shall not exert influence on individuals under his/her care or their families to use products or services based on the direct or indirect financial interest of the physical therapist in such products or services. Realizing that these individuals will normally rely on the physical therapist's advice, their best interest must always be maintained, as must their right of free choice relating to the use of any product or service. Although it cannot be considered unethical for physical therapists to own or have a financial interest in the production, sale, or distribution of products/services, they must act in accordance with law and make full disclosure of their interest whenever individuals under their care use such products/services.

B. A physical therapist may receive remuneration for endorsement or advertisement of products or services to the public, physical therapists, or other health professionals provided he/she discloses any financial interest in the production, sale, or distribution of said products or services.

C. When endorsing or advertising products or services, a physical therapist shall use sound professional judgment and shall not give the appearance of Association endorsement unless the Association has formally endorsed the products or services.

7.3 Disclosure

A physical therapist shall disclose to the patient if the referring practitioner derives compensation from the provision of physical therapy.

Principle 8

A physical therapist shall provide and make available accurate and relevant information to patients/clients about their care and to the public about physical therapy services.

8.1 Accurate and Relevant Information to the Patient

A. A physical therapist shall provide the patient/client accurate and relevant information about his/her condition and plan of care. See Section 2.4.

B. Upon the request of the patient, the physical therapist shall provide, or make available, the medical record to the patient or a patient-designated third party.

C. A physical therapist shall inform patients of any known financial limitations that may affect their care.

D. A physical therapist shall inform the patient when, in his/her judgment, the patient will receive negligible benefit from further care. See Section 7.1.C.

8.2 Accurate and Relevant Information to the Public

A. A physical therapist shall inform the public about the societal benefits of the profession and who is qualified to provide physical therapy services.

B. Information given to the public shall emphasize that individual problems cannot be treated without individualized examination and plans/programs of care.

C. A physical therapist may advertise his/her services to the public. See Section 2.2.

D. A physical therapist shall not use, or participate in the use of, any form of communication containing a false, plagiarized, fraudulent, deceptive, unfair, or sensational statement or claim. See Section 2.2.

E. A physical therapist who places a paid advertisement shall identify it as such unless it is apparent from the context that it is a paid advertisement.

Principle 9

A physical therapist shall protect the public and the profession from unethical, incompetent, and illegal acts.

9.1 Consumer Protection

A. A physical therapist shall provide care that is within the scope of practice as defined by the state practice act.

B. A physical therapist shall not engage in any conduct that is unethical, incompetent or illegal.

C. A physical therapist shall report any conduct that appears to be unethical, incompetent, or illegal.

D. A physical therapist may not participate in any arrangements in which patients are exploited due to the referring sources' enhancing their personal incomes as a result of referring for, prescribing, or recommending physical therapy. See Sections 2.1.B, 4, and 7.

Principle 10

A physical therapist shall endeavor to address the health needs of society.

10.1 Pro Bono Service

A physical therapist shall render pro bono publico (reduced or no fee) services to patients lacking the ability to pay for services, as each physical therapist's practice permits.

10.2 Individual and Community Health

A. A physical therapist shall be aware of the patient's health-related needs and act in a manner that facilitates meeting those needs.

B. A physical therapist shall endeavor to support activities that benefit the health status of the community. See Section 3.

Principle 11

A physical therapist shall respect the rights, knowledge, and skills of colleagues and other health care professionals.

11.1 Consultation

A physical therapist shall seek consultation whenever the welfare of the patient will be safeguarded or advanced by consulting those who have special skills, knowledge, and experience.

11.2 Patient/Provider Relationships

A physical therapist shall not undermine the relationship(s) between his/her patient and other health care professionals.

11.3 Disparagement

Physical therapists shall not disparage colleagues and other health care professionals. See Section 9 and Section 2.4.A.

Issued by Ethics and Judicial Committee
American Physical Therapy Association
October 1981
Last Amended January 2004

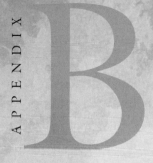

American Physical Therapy Association Standards of Ethical Conduct for the Physical Therapist Assistant and the Guide for Conduct of the Affiliate Member

Standards of Ethical Conduct for the Physical Therapist Assistant

HOD S06 00 13-24 (Program 17)
Amended HOD 06-91-06-07
Initial HOD 06-82-04-08 (Standard)

Preamble

This document of the American Physical Therapy Association sets forth standards for the ethical conduct of the physical therapist assistant. All physical therapist assistants are responsible for maintaining high standards of conduct while assisting physical therapists. The physical therapist assistant shall act in the best interest of the patient/client. These standards of conduct shall be binding on all physical therapist assistants.

Standard 1

A physical therapist assistant shall respect the rights and dignity of all individuals and shall provide compassionate care.

Standard 2

A physical therapist assistant shall act in a trustworthy manner toward patients/clients.

Standard 3

A physical therapist assistant shall provide selected physical therapy interventions only under the supervision and direction of a physical therapist.

Standard 4

A physical therapist assistant shall comply with laws and regulations governing physical therapy.

Standard 5

A physical therapist assistant shall achieve and maintain competence in the provision of selected physical therapy interventions.

Standard 6

A physical therapist assistant shall make judgments that are commensurate with their educational and legal qualifications as a physical therapist assistant.

Standard 7

A physical therapist assistant shall protect the public and the profession from unethical, incompetent, and illegal acts.

Guide for Conduct of the Physical Therapist Assistant

This Guide for Conduct of the Physical Therapist Assistant (Guide) is intended to serve physical therapist assistants in interpreting the Standards of Ethical Conduct for the Physical Therapist Assistant (Standards) of the American Physical Therapy Association (APTA). The Guide provides guidelines by which physical therapist assistants may determine the propriety of their conduct. It is also intended to guide the development of physical therapist assistant students. The Standards and Guide apply to all physical therapist assistants. These guidelines are subject to change as the dynamics of the profession change and as new patterns of health care delivery are developed and accepted by the professional community and the public. This Guide is subject to monitoring and timely revision by the Ethics and Judicial Committee of the Association.

Interpreting Standards

The interpretations expressed in this Guide reflect the opinions, decisions, and advice of the Ethics and Judicial Committee. These interpretations are intended to guide a physical therapist assistant in applying general ethical principles to specific situations. They should not be considered inclusive of all situations that a physical therapist assistant may encounter.

Standard 1

A physical therapist assistant shall respect the rights and dignity of all individuals and shall provide compassionate care.

1.1 Attitude of a Physical Therapist Assistant

A. A physical therapist assistant shall recognize, respect, and respond to individual and cultural difference with compassion and sensitivity.
B. A physical therapist assistant shall be guided at all times by concern for the physical and psychological welfare of patients/clients.
C. A physical therapist assistant shall not harass, abuse, or discriminate against others.

Standard 2

A physical therapist assistant shall act in a trustworthy manner toward patients/clients.

2.1 Trustworthiness

A. The physical therapist assistant shall always place the patients/clients interest(s) above those of the physical therapist assistant. Working in the patient's/client's best interest requires sensitivity to the patient's/client's vulnerability and an effective working relationship between the physical therapist and the physical therapist assistant.

B. A physical therapist assistant shall not exploit any aspect of the physical therapist assistant–patient/client relationship.

C. A physical therapist assistant shall clearly identify himself/herself as a physical therapist assistant to patients/clients.

D. A physical therapist assistant shall conduct himself/herself in a manner that supports the physical therapist–patient/client relationship.

E. A physical therapist assistant shall not engage in any sexual relationship or activity, whether consensual or nonconsensual, with any patient/client entrusted to his/her care.

F. A physical therapist assistant shall not invite, accept, or offer gifts or other considerations that affect or give an appearance of affecting his/her provision of physical therapy interventions. See Section 6.3

2.2 Exploitation of Patients

A physical therapist assistant shall not participate in any arrangements in which patients/clients are exploited. Such arrangements include situations where referring sources enhance their personal incomes by referring to or recommending physical therapy services.

2.3 Truthfulness

A. A physical therapist assistant shall not make statements that he/she knows or should know are false, deceptive, fraudulent, or misleading.

B. Although it cannot be considered unethical for a physical therapist assistant to own or have a financial interest in the production, sale, or distribution of products/services, he/she must act in accordance with law and make full disclosure of his/her interest to patients/clients.

2.4 Confidential Information

A. Information relating to the patient/client is confidential and shall not be communicated to a third party not involved in that patient's/client's care without the prior consent of the patient/client, subject to applicable law.

B. A physical therapist assistant shall refer all requests for release of confidential information to the supervising physical therapist.

Standard 3

A physical therapist assistant shall provide selected physical therapy interventions only under the supervision and direction of a physical therapist.

3.1 Supervisory Relationship

A. A physical therapist assistant shall provide interventions only under the supervision and direction of a physical therapist.
B. A physical therapist assistant shall provide only those interventions that have been selected by the physical therapist.
C. A physical therapist assistant shall not provide any interventions that are outside his/her education, training, experience, or skill and shall notify the responsible physical therapist of his/her inability to carry out the intervention. See Sections 5.1 and 6.1B.
D. A physical therapist assistant may modify specific interventions within the plan of care established by the physical therapist in response to changes in the patient's/client's status.
E. A physical therapist assistant shall not perform examinations and evaluations, determine diagnoses and prognoses, or establish or change a plan of care.
F. Consistent with the physical therapist assistant's education, training, knowledge, and experience, he/she may respond to the patient's/client's inquiries regarding interventions that are within the established plan of care.
G. A physical therapist assistant shall have regular and ongoing communication with the physical therapist regarding the patient's/client's status.

Standard 4

A physical therapist assistant shall comply with laws and regulations governing physical therapy.

4.1 Supervision

A physical therapist assistant shall know and comply with applicable law. Regardless of the content of any law, a physical therapist assistant shall provide services only under the supervision and direction of a physical therapist.

4.2 Representation

A physical therapist assistant shall not hold himself/herself out as a physical therapist.

Standard 5

A physical therapist assistant shall achieve and maintain competence in the provision of selected physical therapy interventions.

5.1 Competence

A physical therapist assistant shall provide interventions consistent with his/her level of education, training, experience, and skill. See Sections 3.1C and 6.1 B.

5.2 Self-assessment

A physical therapist assistant shall engage in self-assessment in order to maintain competence.

5.3 Development

A physical therapist assistant shall participate in educational activities that enhance his/her basic knowledge and skills.

Standard 6

A physical therapist assistant shall make judgments that are commensurate with his/her educational and legal qualifications as a physical therapist assistant.

6.1 Patient Safety

A. A physical therapist assistant shall discontinue immediately any interventions(s) that, in his/her judgment, may be harmful to the patient/client and shall discuss his/her concerns with the physical therapist.
B. A physical therapist assistant shall not provide any interventions that are outside his/her education, training, experience, or skill and shall notify the responsible physical therapist of his/her inability to carry out the intervention. See Sections 3.1C and 5.1.
C. A physical therapist assistant shall not perform interventions while his/her ability to do so safely is impaired.

6.2 Judgments of Patient/Client Status

If, in the judgment of the physical therapist assistant, there is a change in the patient/client status, he/she shall report this to the responsible physical therapist. See Section 3.1.

6.3 Gifts and Other Considerations

A physical therapist assistant shall not invite, accept, or offer gifts, monetary incentives, or other considerations that affect or give an appearance of affecting his/her provision of physical therapy interventions. See Section 2.1F.

Standard 7

A physical therapist assistant shall protect the public and the profession from unethical, incompetent, and illegal acts.

7.1 Consumer Protection

A physical therapist assistant shall report any conduct that appears to be unethical or illegal.

7.2 Organizational Employment

A. A physical therapist assistant shall inform his/her employer(s) and/or appropriate physical therapist of any employer practice that causes him or her to be in conflict with the Standards of Ethical Conduct for the Physical Therapist Assistant.

B. A physical therapist assistant shall not engage in any activity that puts him or her in conflict with the Standards of Ethical Conduct for the Physical Therapist Assistant, regardless of directives from a physical therapist or employer.

———

Issued by Ethics and Judicial Committee
American Physical Therapy Association
October 1981
Last Amended February 2004

Preventing Sexual Harassment in the Workplace: A Sample Policy and Complaint Procedure

Table of Contents

Introduction

For the past several years, both public awareness of inappropriate behavior and substantial court awards have resulted in an increase in sexual harassment complaints filed by either direct victims or persons working in a hostile work environment.

Sexual harassment occurs frequently in office situations, and [physical therapy practices] are no exceptions. Serious professionalism questions may be raised when sexual harassment and other forms of discrimination are shown to exist.

Sexual harassment is a form of discrimination on the basis of gender. Sexual harassment violates federal civil rights statutes, as well as various state and local statutes. The principal federal statute, Title VII of the Civil Rights Act of 1964, as amended, 42 U.S.C.A. Sections 2000e, et seq., 2000e-2(a)(1), applies to [businesses] with 15 or more employees (not including partners in a true partnership). State statutes or local ordinances may apply to [smaller businesses].

If your [business] is not subject to any statute or ordinance, issuing a policy may give your employees more contractual rights than they otherwise would have. Even if the statutes do not currently cover your situation, there are additional factors for you to consider when deciding whether to implement a policy against sexual harassment:

A. Even if your [business] is not subject to statutory law, an employee claiming sexual harassment in the terms and conditions of employment may have valid tort claims, including assault and battery, wrongful discharge, or intentional infliction of emotional distress. Adoption of a policy accompanied with training should be helpful in avoiding the conduct, which could give rise to a tort claim.

B. Disciplinary Rule 1-102B does address the possibility of sexual harassment, together with other discriminatory conduct in a physical therapist's dealings with clients and employees, rising to the level of unethical conduct. If so, sanctions would be a possibility.

C. An employer which permits either a hostile work environment to exist, or treats employees more or less favorably for reasons relating to actual sexual relationships, will adversely affect both the morale and the productivity of the workplace.

A [business] should weigh all of these factors when deciding whether to adopt a policy and educate [business] members and staff about the problems of sexual harassment.

Generally, sexual harassment takes one of two forms: (1) quid pro quo or (2) hostile environment. In quid pro quo sexual harassment, the terms and conditions of employment are expressly linked to the employee's engaging in sexual conduct. In hostile environment harassment, repeated unwanted sexual gestures, jokes, overtures, touching, and the like create a hostile work environment for one or more employees. It is not only the "harasser" who can be held responsible. The doctrine of respondeat superior may be applicable. In a small [business] setting, it would be more difficult to establish that sexual harassment occurred without the managing physical therapist's awareness.

The sample policy that follows has been carefully drafted but should not be adopted thoughtlessly. What works for a large [business] may not work for a small [business]. For example, the requirement of a committee investigation or the provision concerning an alternative person to whom a situation may be reported should be based on your [business]'s structure. Confidentiality can also be a concern from both the accuser's and the accused's points of view. What works for another [business] of your identical size may not work for yours. In a partnership form of business, one partner's knowledge of certain conduct may be imputed to other partners. You must tailor the policy to fit the [business]. Further, the adoption of a policy should not be your final step. Education of [business] members and employees and integration of the policy with your existing procedures on maintenance of personnel files and their confidences are also important. Finally, we want you to know that there are qualified mediators available, for a fee, to mediate sexual harassment claims.

The sample policy is not intended to establish a minimum standard of care, nor does it represent a legal defense to any claims of sexual harassment. The sample policy should not be considered either the practice of law or providing legal advice. This document is intended to make practitioners aware of the issues and to suggest ways to handle some issues without litigation. Be advised that the law can change at any time.

Preventing Sexual Harassment in the [Physical Therapy] Workplace: A Sample Policy

A. Statement of [Business] Philosophy
([BUSINESS] NAME) is committed to maintaining a professional and collegial work environment in which all individuals are treated with respect and dignity. Each individual has the right to work in a professional atmosphere that promotes equal opportunities and prohibits discriminatory practices, including sexual harassment. At ([BUSINESS] NAME), sexual harassment, whether verbal, physical, or arising out of the work assignments at the office, at office-sponsored social functions, or elsewhere, is unacceptable and will not be tolerated. It is also illegal.

B. Definition of Sexual Harassment
For purposes of this policy, *sexual harassment* is defined as unwelcome and unwanted sexual advances, requests for sexual favors, and other verbal, nonverbal, or physical conduct of a sexual nature when (1) submission to or rejection of this conduct by an individual is used explicitly or implicitly as a factor in decisions affecting hiring, evaluation, promotion, or other aspects of employment; or (2) this conduct substantially interferes with an individual's employment or creates an intimidating, hostile or offensive work environment.

Examples of sexual harassment include, but are not limited to, unwanted sexual advances; demands for sexual favors in exchange for favorable treatment or continued employment; repeated sexual jokes, flirtations, advances, or propositions; verbal abuse of a sexual nature; graphic, verbal commentary about an individual's body, sexual prowess, or sexual deficiencies; leering; whistling; touching; pinching; assault; coerced sexual acts; suggestive insulting, obscene comments or gestures; and display in the workplace of sexually suggestive objects or pictures.

This behavior is unacceptable in the workplace itself and by any owner, partner, or employee in any business-related setting outside the workplace, including but not limited to other work-related settings such as business trips, court appearances, and business-related social events.

(The [business] may also want to consider placing a "fraternization" warning here that would state, "Consenting romantic and sexual relationships between members and/or employees of the [business] are not expressly forbidden, but such relationships are considered very unwise because factors such as real or perceived power of one person over another within the [business] may override claims of consent at a later date.")

C. Individuals Covered by the Policy

This policy covers all employees ([physical therapists, physical therapist assistants, aides, administrative staff]). ([BUSINESS] NAME) will not tolerate sexual harassment, whether engaged in by fellow employees, supervisors, or associates, or by other non-employees who conduct business with this [business]. In addition, the [business] will not tolerate sexual harassment engaged in by an individual who is not an employee of the [business] (e.g., patient, vendor, patient family member]) to the extent that it affects any employee of the [business]. Any employee who has been subject to sexual harassment by such a person may complain to (THE [BUSINESS]'S APPOINTED COMMITTEE OR ANY MEMBER THEREOF). (If a "committee" is not practical for the [business], an individual from within or without the [business] could be designated. Similar changes in the sample policy would be necessary to accommodate the needs of the [business]). The [business] will investigate any incident of alleged sexual harassment by a person who is not an employee of the [business] to the extent practical and will take any action it deems appropriate after evaluating all the circumstances. In particular with respect to patients, the [business] will take any action necessary to stop the conduct, and, if not stopped, the [business] will terminate its relationship with the patient, if appropriate. The [business] encourages reporting of all incidents of sexual harassment, regardless of who the offender may be, in accordance with the method set out in Section D.

D. How to Report a Complaint

1. Informal Procedure

([BUSINESS] NAME) encourages individuals who believe they are being harassed to clearly and promptly notify the offender that his or her behavior is unwelcome. If for any reason an individual does not wish to approach the offender directly or if such discussion does not successfully end the harassment, then the individual should notify a member of (THE [BUSINESS]'S APPOINTED COMMITTEE) [as described below] who may talk to the alleged harasser or arrange for mediation between the individual and the alleged harasser with a third person acceptable to both. This informal procedure is not a required first step for the reporting individual.

2. Formal Procedure.

In the event that the reporting individual does not wish to pursue the informal procedure, or in the event that the informal procedure does not produce a result satisfactory to the reporting individual, the following steps should be followed to report the sexual harassment complaint and to initiate a formal procedure:

a. Notification of a Member of the Staff.

An individual who believes he or she has been subject to sexual harassment should report the incident to any member of (THE [BUSINESS]'S APPOINTED COMMITTEE). The current members of the committee are (list names). (The [business] should designate more than one individual within the [business] to receive complaints. To the extent feasible, these individuals should reflect the diversity of the [business], in gender, as well as age and seniority).

An individual also has the option of reporting the harassment to the individual's supervisor. In such a case, the supervisor must immediately file a written report of the complaint and its resolution with a member of (THE [BUSINESS]'S APPOINTED COMMITTEE).

Any investigation should be confidential to ensure the privacy of the persons involved. Both the accuser and accused individuals should be reminded of the confidential nature of the process.

b. Description of Misconduct

An accurate record of objectionable behavior is necessary to resolve a formal complaint of sexual harassment. All complaints of sexual harassment must be reduced to writing by either the reporting individual or the individual(s) designated to receive complaints.

c. Time for Reporting a Complaint

Prompt reporting of complaints is strongly encouraged because it allows for rapid response and resolution of objectionable behavior or conditions for the reporting individual and any other affected employees. This [business] has chosen not to impose a limited time frame for the reporting of sexual harassment complaints. However, the reporting individual should be aware that applicable statutes of limitations do constrain the time for instituting outside legal action.

d. Protection Against Retaliation

This [business] will not retaliate against an individual who makes a report of sexual harassment, nor permit any employee to do so. Retaliation is a very serious violation of this policy and should be reported immediately. Any individual found to have retaliated against an individual for reporting sexual harassment, or against anyone participating in the investigation of a complaint, will be subject to appropriate disciplinary procedures as described below. (See "How to Resolve the Complaint.")

E. How to Investigate the Formal Complaint

1. Confidentiality

Any allegation of sexual harassment brought to the attention of (THE [BUSINESS]'S APPOINTED COMMITTEE) will be promptly investigated. Confidentiality will be maintained throughout the investigatory process to the extent practical and appropriate under the circumstances.

2. Identification of Investigators

Complaints will be initially investigated by the person on (THE [BUSINESS]'S APPOINTED COMMITTEE) to whom it was reported, unless the committee determines another person should be the investigator.

3. Investigation Process

The investigation process may include any or all of the following:
- Confirm name and position of the reporting individual.
- Identify the alleged harasser.
- Thoroughly ascertain all facts in connection with the alleged incident, beginning by interviewing the reporting individual and the alleged harasser. Questions of all parties should be asked in a nonjudgmental manner.
- Determine frequency/type of alleged harassment and, if possible, the dates and locations where alleged harassment occurred.
- Find out if any witness observed the alleged harassment. If the reporting individual and the alleged harasser present conflicting versions of the facts, interview any witnesses.
- Ask how the reporting individual responded to the alleged harassment, and determine what efforts, if any, at informal resolution of the matter were made.
- Determine whether the reporting individual consulted anyone else about the alleged harassment, and take note of who else knows and their response to the disclosure.
- Develop a thorough understanding of the professional relationship, degree of control, and amount of interaction between the alleged harasser and reporting individual.
- Determine whether the reporting individual knows of or suspects that there are other individuals who have been harassed by the alleged harasser.
- Determine whether the reporting individual informed supervisors of the situation and what response, if any, reporting individual received from these individuals.
- During the first interview with the alleged harasser, remind the alleged harasser of the [business]'s policy against retaliation for making a complaint of sexual harassment.

In pursuing the investigation, the investigator will try to take the wishes of the reporting individual into consideration, but he or she should thoroughly investigate the matter, keeping both parties informed as to the status of the investigation.

F. How to Resolve the Complaint

Upon completing the investigation, the investigator will report to (THE [BUSINESS]'S APPOINTED COMMITTEE). (THE [BUSINESS]'S APPOINTED COMMITTEE) will review the investigation, make findings and decide upon appropriate action to be taken. (THE [BUSINESS]'S APPOINTED COMMITTEE) will communicate its findings and intended actions to the reporting individual and alleged harasser.

If (THE [BUSINESS]'S APPOINTED COMMITTEE) finds that harassment occurred, the harasser will be subject to appropriate disciplinary procedures, as listed in the following sections.

1. Sanctions for Harassment

Individuals found to have engaged in misconduct constituting sexual harassment shall be disciplined. Appropriate sanctions will be determined by (SELECT THE APPROPRIATE INDIVIDUAL OR GROUP OF INDIVIDUALS). In addressing incidents of sexual harassment, the [business]'s response at a minimum will include reprimanding the offender and preparing a written record. Additional action may include the following: referral to counseling, withholding of a promotion, reassignment, temporary suspension without pay, reduction in allocation, discharge, or removal or expulsion from the [business].

2. False Accusations

If an investigation results in a finding that the reporting individual falsely and maliciously accused another of sexual harassment, the reporting individual will be subject to appropriate sanctions, as described above, including the possibility of termination.

G. Appeals Process

If either party directly involved in a sexual harassment investigation is dissatisfied with the outcome or resolution, that individual has the right to appeal the decision. The dissatisfied party should submit written comments in a timely manner to (SELECT THE APPROPRIATE REVIEWERS; INDIVIDUAL OR GROUP; E.G. [CLINICAL MANAGER], ETC.).

The (APPEALS COMMITTEE) will review the objecting party's position and the entire record before it and present its findings within _____ calendar days of receiving the written objection.

H. Maintaining a Written Record of the Complaint

([BUSINESS] NAME) shall maintain a complete written record of each complaint and how it was investigated and resolved. Written records shall be maintained in a confidential manner to the extent practical and appropriate in the office of (NAME THE APPROPRIATE INDIVIDUAL OR APPROPRIATE DIVISION WITHIN THE OFFICE). (The keeper of the records may vary depending on who filed the complaint.)

I. Mediation (Optional)

As an alternative for those wishing to resolve disputes among themselves without resorting to this policy, we will, if all parties agree, make available a trained outside mediator to help you find an amicable, informal solution. If mediation does not solve the problem, you may still use the procedures in this policy.

J. Conclusion

([BUSINESS] NAME) has developed this policy to ensure that all of its employees can work in an environment free from sexual harassment. This policy will be immediately disseminated to all employees, and the [business] will provide this policy to all new employees upon their arrival at the [business]. (THE [BUSINESS]'S APPOINTED COMMITTEE) will conduct informational sessions concerning the policy so as to ensure that all employees understand the [business]'s commitment to eliminating any sexual harassment in the work place, are familiar with the policy and know that any complaint received will be investigated and appropriately resolved.

Adapted from Ohio State Bar Association: *Sexual harassment in the legal workplace,* For Ohio Law Firms, June 1998.

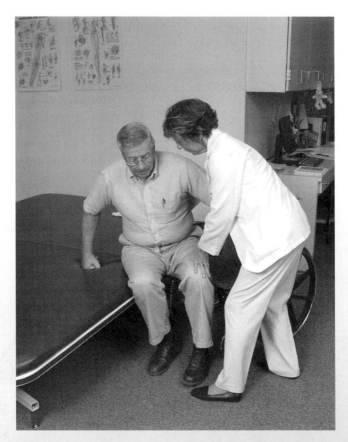

From Pierson F, Fairchild S: *Principles and techniques of patient care in physical therapy,* ed 4, St Louis, 2008, Saunders.

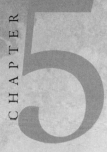

CHAPTER 5

Information, Quality, and Risk Management

Ron Scott

ABSTRACT

The effective and efficient simultaneous management of patient care and related information, high-quality health care service delivery, and liability risk exposure are crucial to successful clinical management. No other areas of clinical management are as heavily law focused and regulation laden as are these practice areas. Physical therapy clinical managers must consult regularly and proactively with legal counsel to stay abreast of federal, state, and local laws and regulations concerning such issues as compliance with regulatory and statutory pronouncements; the generation, disposition, and legal status of incident reports; malpractice case law pronouncements and liability trends; and privacy issues involving protected health information (PHI), among many other related topics. This chapter explores key issues in these areas, offering selected case examples and sample formats for adaptation by readers, in consultation with their legal counsel, staffs, and administrators.

KEY WORDS AND PHRASES

Commission on
  Accreditation of
  Rehabilitation Facilities
  (CARF)
Communication
Electronic Signatures in
  Global and National
  Commerce Act
Health care malpractice
Health Insurance
  Portability and
  Accountability
  Act (HIPAA)

Improvement of organiza-
  tional performance
Incident reporting
Information management
Information management
  systems
Liability
National Committee for
  Quality Assurance
  (NCQA)
Privacy
Professional liability
  insurance

Quality
Quality management
Risk management
Telehealth
Telemedicine
The Joint Commission
  (TJC)
Uniform Electronic
  Transactions Act

OBJECTIVES

1. Identify the formidable legal and ethical duties incumbent upon clinical health care managers and providers related to the generation, maintenance, and dissemination of health-related information.

2. Provide examples of ways in which health care information management is highly complex and subject to substantial legal, regulatory, and accreditation oversight.

3. Understand the primary reason that care providers document patient care activities and discuss the ways in which these professionals communicate important care-related information about patients and clients to other health care professionals.

4. Practice effective documentation risk management so as to protect against breaches of patient confidentiality and record spoliation.

5. Carry out appropriate and effective adverse incident reporting in physical therapy clinical practice.

6. Apply the panoply of quality management tools in clinical practice so as to optimize high-quality physical therapy clinical health care delivery.

7. Educate patients about their shared responsibility for high-quality care delivery through the development and posting of a clinic-specific statement of patient rights and responsibilities.

8. Exercise all reasonable and prudent preventive steps to avoid allegations of harm to patients in the course of physical therapy care delivery.

9. Evaluate, in consultation with legal counsel, the relative merits in obtaining and maintaining individual professional liability insurance in order to transfer the risk of monetary loss incident to health care malpractice to providers' insurers.

10. Synthesize patient-focused quality management and self-protective risk management into a unitary clinical practice standard that simultaneously optimizes quality patient care delivery and minimizes provider liability risk exposure.

MANAGEMENT OF HEALTH CARE INFORMATION

One of the most formidable legal and ethical duties incumbent upon clinical health care managers and providers is the compliant generation, maintenance, and appropriate dissemination of health-related information.[23] Clinical managers have primary responsibility for managing not only patient care–related information but also business-oriented information, much of which is proprietary and subject to limited or nonpublic release.

Information management is complex and subject to substantial legal, regulatory, and accreditation oversight.[29] Computerized **information management systems** complement and, in some cases, have overtaken paper record management systems in health care organizations. Many health care organizations and systems have converted completely to integrated computerized information management networks.[42]

In addition to the advantages of quicker, easier **communication** of vital patient information and documentation of care rendered (after overcoming the computer learning curve), certain adjunctive disadvantages characterize computerized information systems and networks, particularly **privacy** concerns.[27] Such systems feature elaborate security features to minimize the risk of disclosure of confidential patient and business information to unauthorized parties.[25]

New and developing statutory and administrative agency laws and regulations promise to change the landscape of patient care documentation, including the recently implemented federal **Health Insurance Portability and Accountability Act (HIPAA)** regulations, promulgated by the Department of Health and Human Services.[6,33,40] Its attention to private, protected patient health information should provide guidance for drafters of another pending federal statute, addressing electronic medical records, which may label patient electronic medical information "proprietary."[4]

Patient care documentation serves a myriad of important health-related, business, legal, and ethical purposes. The primary reason that primary health care providers document their examinations, evaluations, diagnoses, prognoses, interventions, and referrals is to communicate important care-related information about patients and clients to other health care professionals who have a legitimate official need for the information provided.[31,35]

Communication, then, is the principle reason underlying documentation and information management. Obviously, the most critically important communications involve emergent patient care information transmitted to other health care providers with co-responsibilities for the care of such patients. All other purposes for documenting patient care activities—from creating a record for reimbursement[3,5,8,16,33] to creating a legal record or a historical record for peer review, quality improvement activities, and research—are of secondary importance. It is a form of professional negligence (which becomes legally actionable **health care malpractice** if a patient suffers resultant injury) to fail to document patient care–related findings and activities in a timely manner and in a form that is accurate, clear, comprehensive, concise, and objective.[11] The 2006 CNA Physical Therapy Claims Study cited the failure to appropriately communicate patients' conditions to referring physicians and others as the primary reason for the most costly (severe) claims payouts.[31]

Information security processes involving computerized patient care documentation effectively protect against breaches of patient confidentiality and spoliation (or impermissible alteration or destruction of patient care records to hide their meaning) by limiting access to authorized system users and by disallowing the substitution of altered record entries for original ones.

Laws, such as the **Uniform Electronic Transactions Act** and the 2000 **Electronic Signatures in Global and National Commerce Act**, have made electronic and digital signatures nearly universally acceptable in business transactions (including health care).[20] The specific language of the Electronic Signatures Act is purposefully vague regarding the parameters of an electronic signature, leaving relatively wide latitude for developing convenient system-specific models on an individual basis. Clinic managers should consult with legal counsel before implementing such a system.

Electronic data transfer and the universal acceptance of electronic signatures may lead to expanded virtual health care delivery in the not-too-distant future. **Telemedicine** (involving physician intervention with patients) and **telehealth** (involving physician and nonphysician health care professionals) offer great benefits to patients and providers, including universal access to health care services; diminished pain and suffering on the part of patients who would otherwise wait for, or not receive, care; and time efficiency and safety for providers.[20,22] Telehealth also carries with it substantial risks of possible harm to patients, providers, and the integrity of the system, including illegal and unethical breaches of confidentiality of patient information,[1,2,17,34] possible derogation from the heretofore close professional relationship between patients and providers, and provider **liability** for unlicensed practice across state lines. Careful, thorough, secure patient care documentation is a requisite to providing telehealth services.[4] Other legal, administrative, and sociocultural issues associated with telehealth have yet to be satisfactorily addressed.

EXERCISE **5-1**

Brainstorm to create a list of at least 10 ways that clinical physical therapists may be able to deliver telehealth patient care services over the Internet now or in the near future. What impediments other than indirect physical therapist-patient contact hinder development and effectiveness of such endeavors? How, if at all, can these impediments be overcome?

Patients are savvy customers who increasingly know and exercise their legal rights, including the right of direct access to their medical records. Many patients keep elaborate informal ambulatory backup records of their own care, often storing such information on Internet sites that store health-related information for clients.[19]

Patient Privacy

Patient privacy is a seminal issue in clinical health care delivery. Similarly, no issue in health care clinical management carries with it such profound legal and ethical issues as patient health care information management and the safeguarding of private patient information. The potential adverse consequences of an impermissible breach of patient privacy for the patient, the patient's family and significant others, providers, and the health care clinic and organization make its safeguarding a critically important management issue. The federal HIPAA privacy and security rules, applicable to a broad range of health care providers and organizations and discussed in greater detail later in this chapter, make patient information privacy management more manageable, although also administratively burdensome.[14]

Information privacy has been a spearhead issue in the late twentieth and early twenty-first centuries.[12] The fundamental trust in the legal and medical systems themselves turns in large part on the confidentiality of private information shared by patients with their providers.[10] The nearly inviolable nature of the attorney-client, and to a lesser degree, the health care professional-patient relationship, facilitates this free exchange of vital information between professionals and clients.

Before recent legal cases, statutes, regulations, and expansion of individual privacy protections under the federal Constitution, privacy was only a relatively obscure common law issue, for the breach of which an unauthorized discloser of private facts about patients merely faced civil liability for invasion of privacy. Only in 1965 did the federal government, through the Congress and the United States Supreme Court, definitively address medical privacy. In the landmark initial privacy law case of *Griswold v. Connecticut*, the United States Supreme Court ruled for the first time that a newly created federal constitutional right of privacy permitted couples to purchase and use contraceptives for birth control within the marital relationship.

The Court in *Griswold* created what is the only unwritten, or implicit, individual right under the Bill of Rights—that is, the constitutional right of privacy. However, because the individual liberties delineated in the Bill of Rights apply only to governmental action (except for the Thirteenth Amendment, which addresses slavery and involuntary servitude generally), individual privacy is constitutionally protected only from federal, state, and local governmental intrusion. Therefore only clinicians within state or federal health facilities are covered by its provisions and restrictions. Other federal, state, and local laws protect individuals from unwarranted nongovernmental privacy intrusions, such as wiretap and credit reporting statutes and regulations.

In the same year that the Court decided *Griswold*, Congress enacted Medicare and Medicaid and made patient information privacy an express condition of participation by providers and facilities in these programs, which today account for nearly half of third-party-payer funding of health care services.

Other laws augmented federal and state privacy laws and case decisions over the next quarter century, including, but certainly not limited to, *Roe v. Wade* (1973, abortion), the federal Privacy Act and Family Education Rights and Privacy Act (1974), federal Protection of Human Subjects Regulations (1979), the Electronic Communications Privacy Act (1979, addressing email privacy), the Health Insurance Portability and Accountability Act (HIPAA, 1996), and Executive Order 13145 (2000, prohibiting the use of genetic history or information in federal employment).

Patient informed consent to health care intervention is perhaps the most advanced manifestation of respect for individual autonomy and privacy. Physical therapists, like all clinical health care professionals, must make adequate disclosure of relevant care-related information to patients (or their surrogate decision makers) to enable them to make informed decisions about whether to accept or reject recommended care plans. Patient informed consent policies and procedure should require written, patient-signed informed consent for high-risk, invasive, or peri-operative interventions, or whenever patients are in active litigation.[31,37]

Health Insurance Portability and Accountability Act

HIPAA has two broad purposes: to facilitate the transferability of employee health insurance benefits between public and private-sector jobs and to safeguard the sanctity and privacy of individual protected health information (PHI).[38] Because Congress procrastinated and did not enact enabling privacy legislation by August 1999, the Department of Health and Human Services went on to create and implement privacy regulations pursuant to HIPAA. After the required comment period, these regulations became law on April 14, 2001, with an effective date of April 23, 2003. Shortly after its effective date, President George W. Bush made patient informed consent to information dissemination voluntary and oral, instead of mandatory, as the original legislation required. At a recent meeting of the American Health Care Lawyers Association, Department of Health and Human Services officials estimated that health care providers' and organizations' administrative burdens under the HIPAA privacy rules would increase by up to 25%.[32,44]

The privacy rules do several important things for patients. They afford them greater autonomy over private health data. They also set strict limits on how individual health information is gathered, stored, and released by health care providers and organizations, holding covered providers and health care organizations legally accountable for impermissible breaches of patient privacy. Informed consent, albeit not necessarily in writing, is a prerequisite for the use or dissemination of PHI for purposes of treatment, payment, or operations (TPO).

Health care systems, plans, providers, and clearinghouses that conduct financial transactions electronically must be committed to compliance with the letter and spirit of HIPAA in receiving, processing, storing, transmitting, and otherwise handling PHI.

HIPAA's privacy standards represent the first comprehensive federal guidelines for protection of PHI. Supplemental guidance and protections are found in state and local case law, statutes, and administrative rules and regulations. Protection extends to any individually identifiable health information, maintained or transmitted in any medium, held by any covered entity or business associate of a covered entity.

Covered entities must also obtain adequate contractual assurances from business associates that the latter will appropriately safeguard patient PHI that comes to them. Examples of activities that may be conducted by business associates include benefit management, billing, claims processing, data analysis, quality improvement management, practice management, and utilization review. If a business associate is found to have violated HIPAA, the covered entity must first attempt to "cure" (correct) the breach (violation) of contract and, if unsuccessful, terminate the contract with the noncompliant business associate and report the matter to the Secretary of the Department of Health and Human Services for possible administrative action.

Each employee, contractor, and consultant is a fiduciary, owing a personal duty to patients to take all reasonable steps pursuant to HIPAA to safeguard their PHI. All employees and other providers must receive HIPAA training during initial orientation and periodically thereafter to update their knowledge of HIPAA.

Providers and entities covered by HIPAA must exercise reasonable caution under all circumstances to disclose only the minimum necessary amount of PHI in order to comply with their legal duties owed to patients and others.

On the first visit to any covered provider, all patients must be made aware of the facility's HIPAA Privacy Policy. Direct care providers must issue a Patient Notice of Privacy Practices to all patients at first contact and make a good-faith attempt to obtain their written acknowledgment of receipt of the document. In addition, providers must post their entire Patient Notice of Privacy Practices in their facility in a prominent location for patient to see. Examples of HIPAA Patient Notice of Privacy Practices documents in English and Spanish appear in Appendices A and B.

Normally, a covered entity (any provider filing reimbursement claims electronically) may use and disclose a patient's PHI for purposes of treatment, payment for services, and internal health care operations of the business without the patient's authorization or consent. These disclosures are called *routine uses.*

Regarding patient informed consent for routine uses of PHI, providers are required only to make a good faith effort to obtain informed consent for treatment, payment, and health care operations. Covered entities have wide discretion to design processes that mesh with their individual practices. Patients have the right to request restrictions on the use or disclosure of their PHI, but covered entities are not required to agree to such restrictions.

There are three general classifications of PHI disclosures under HIPAA: permissive and mandatory (both without patient authorization or consent), and authorized. Permissive disclosures include those necessary for TPO. This includes, among other possibilities, communication between and among treatment team members, determination of coverage for health services, and peer/utilization review activities.

Required disclosures are those made pursuant to legal mandates, such as a court order or state reporting statutes for suspected abuse; communicable diseases, including sexually transmitted diseases; and gunshot wounds. Authorized disclosures encompass broad disclosure authority pursuant to valid written and signed patient authorization.

Regarding minors' PHI, the Privacy Rule generally allows a parent to have access to the medical records about his or her child as the minor child's personal representative, when such access is not inconsistent with state or other laws. There are three situations in which the parent would not be the minor's personal representative under the Privacy Rule. These exceptions are (1) when the minor is the one who consents to care and the consent of the parent is not required under State or other applicable law (e.g., when the minor is emancipated); (2) when the minor obtains care at the direction of a court or a person appointed by the court; and (3) when, and to the extent that, the parent agrees that the minor and the health care provider may have a confidential relationship. However, even in these exceptional situations, the parent may have access to the health record of the minor related to this treatment when state or other applicable law requires or permits such parental access.

Suggested standard operating procedures for clinics that are covered entities under HIPAA's Privacy Rule appear here in a special feature box. The list is not intended to be comprehensive. In addition to appointing and adequately training a clinic privacy officer, the staffs of covered entities should brainstorm to generate lists of standard operating procedures to be implemented for their individual practices.

Providers covered by HIPAA may still use sign-in sheets for patients and clients and call out their names in waiting rooms as long as PHI is not disclosed in these processes.

Standard Operating Procedures Pursuant to HIPAA's Privacy Rule

1. Staff will not allow patient records to be placed or to remain in open (public) view.
2. Staff will not discuss patient protected health information (PHI) within the hearing/perceptive range of third parties not involved in the patient's care.
3. Patients and other non-employees/contractors/consultants are not permitted access to the patient records room.
4. Except where authorized, permitted, or required by law, PHI disclosures require HIPAA-compliant written patient/client authorizations and written requests by requestors for information.
5. Patient records may not be removed from the facility, except for transit to and from secure storage, or otherwise as authorized, permitted, or required by law.
6. Written requests by patients for their health records will be expeditiously honored.
7. Patient records may be placed in chart holders for clinic providers, provided that the following reasonable and appropriate measures are taken to protect the patient's privacy: limiting access to patient care areas and escorting non-employees in the area, ensuring that the areas are supervised, and placing patient/client charts in chart holders with the front cover facing the wall rather than having PHI about the patient visible to anyone who walks by.
8. Providers may leave phone messages for patients on their answering machines. Limit the amount of information disclosed on the answering machine to clinic name and number and any other information necessary to confirm an appointment, asking the individual to call back. It is permissible to leave a similar message with a family member or other person who answers the phone when the patient is not home.
9. The clinic is required to give notice of its privacy policy to every individual receiving treatment no later than the date of first service delivery and to make a good faith effort to obtain the individual's written acknowledgment of receipt of the notice.
10. The clinic also must post its entire privacy policy in the facility in a clear and prominent location where individuals are likely to see it, as well as make the notice available to those who ask for a copy. Copies of the clinic privacy notice are maintained in English and Spanish.

Being seen in a waiting room and hearing one's name called constitute incidental disclosures that do not violate HIPAA, according to the Department of Health and Human Services. A sign-in sheet may not, however, list diagnoses.

Providers may also transmit patient health records to other providers without patient authorization or consent if the new providers are treating the patients for the same conditions as the sending providers. This includes transfer of an entire patient health record (including documentation created by other providers), if reasonably necessary for treatment.

Providers are not normally required to document a disclosure history unless patient authorization is required for disclosure; however, it would be prudent risk management to create and maintain such a history. What is required is that covered providers and entities exercise reasonable caution under all circumstances to disclose only the minimal necessary amount of PHI to comply with their legal duties owed to patients and others.

The HIPAA Privacy Rule does not apply to entities that are workers' compensation insurers, administrative agencies, or employers, except to the extent they may otherwise be covered entities. These entities need access to the health information of individuals who are injured on the job or who have a work-related illness to process and adjudicate claims and to coordinate care under workers' compensation systems. Generally, this health information is obtained from health care providers who are covered by the Privacy Rule.

The Privacy Rule recognizes the legitimate need of insurers and other entities involved in the workers' compensation systems to have access to individuals' health information as authorized by state or other laws. Due to the significant variability among such laws, the Privacy Rule permits disclosures of health information for workers' compensation purposes in a number of different ways.

1. Disclosures without individual authorization. The Privacy Rule permits covered entities to disclose PHI to workers' compensation insurers, state administrators, employers, and other persons or entities involved in workers' compensation systems without the individual's authorization:

    a. As authorized by and to the extent necessary to comply with laws relating to workers' compensation or similar programs established by law that provide benefits for work-related injuries or illness without regard to fault. This includes programs established by the Black Lung Benefits Act, the Federal Employees' Compensation Act, the Longshore and Harbor Workers' Compensation Act, and the Energy Employees' Occupational Illness Compensation Program Act. See 45 CFR 164.512(l).

    b. To the extent the disclosure is required by state or other law. The disclosure must comply with and be limited to what the law requires. See 45 CFR 164.512(a).

    c. For purposes of obtaining payment for any health care provided to the injured or ill worker. See 45 CFR 164.502(a)(1)(ii) and the definition of *payment* at 45 CFR 164.501.

2. Disclosures with individual authorization. In addition, covered entities may disclose PHI to workers' compensation insurers and others involved in workers' compensation systems wherein the individual has provided his or her authorization for the release of the information to the entity. The authorization must contain the elements and otherwise meet the requirements specified at 45 CFR 164.508.

3. Minimum Necessary. Consistent with HIPAA's Privacy Rule main theme, covered entities are required reasonably to limit the amount of PHI disclosed under 45 CFR 164.512(l) to the minimum necessary to accomplish the workers' compensation purpose. Under this requirement, PHI may be shared for such purposes to the full extent authorized by state or other law. In addition, covered entities are required reasonably to limit the amount of PHI disclosed for payment purposes to the minimum necessary. Covered entities are permitted to disclose the amount and types of protected health information that are necessary to obtain payment for health care provided to an injured or ill worker. Where a covered entity routinely makes disclosures for workers' compensation purposes under 45 CFR 164.512(l) or for payment purposes, the covered entity may develop standard protocols as part of its minimum necessary policies and procedures that address the type and amount of protected health information to be disclosed for such purposes. Where protected health information is requested by a state workers' compensation or other public official, covered entities are permitted to reasonably rely on the official's representations that the information requested is the minimum necessary for the intended purpose. See 45 CFR 164.514(d)(3)(iii)(A). Covered entities are not required to make a minimum necessary determination when disclosing PHI as required by state or other law or pursuant to the individual's authorization. See 45 CFR 164.502(b).

HIPAA-related patient complaints should first be directed to an organization's HIPAA privacy officer. A complaint may also be filed with the Office of Civil Rights, U.S. Department of Health and Human Services (DHHS; Box 5-1).

BOX **5-1** ▪ **Department of Health and Human Services Requirements for a Written HIPAA Complaint**

1. Complainant's full name and residential and email addresses, home and work phone numbers
2. Name, address, and phone number of entity violating complainant's protected health information (PHI)
3. Description of the PHI violation
4. Complainant's signature and date
5. Necessary reasonable accommodations, as applicable

An alleged PHI violator is prohibited from taking retaliatory action against a complainant. Potential sanctions for HIPAA Privacy Rule violations include civil and criminal penalties. Civil penalties of between $100 and $25,000 per violation are enforced by the Office of Civil Rights, Department of Health and Human Services. Criminal sanctions of 1 to 10 years' imprisonment and $50,000 to $250,000 fines are enforced by the Department of Justice.

Incident Reporting

The primary purpose for creating and maintaining patient care documentation is to expeditiously communicate important patient information to other health care providers with a legitimate need to know the information conveyed.

Appropriate and effective adverse **incident reporting** is a critically important liability risk management tool.[7,28,36] Incident reports should be properly generated when a patient, staff member, visitor, or other person (or animal) is injured; when a patient expresses serious dissatisfaction with care delivery or care personnel; and when a crime or breach of security occurs on premises.

Normally, incident reports are considered to be private, privileged documents under law, meaning that they are exempt from release to any third parties without the health care organization's consent. Incident reports are, like financial documents, proprietary to health care business organizations and their staffs.

On advice of legal counsel, incident reports should be prominently labeled as quality improvement or attorney work-product documents (or both) to be protected from outside release. Incident reports must contain factual information that is accurate and objective and that is written, whenever possible, by percipient witnesses to adverse events.

The following guidance must be followed. Never speculate as to the cause of an adverse incident, nor assign blame to anyone for an adverse event. Leave that to investigators after the incident report is expeditiously hand-carried to the facility risk manager for processing. If health care professionals are involved as potential defendants in an adverse incident, then report that fact immediately to the institutional risk manager and to the providers so that they may contact their personal attorneys and **professional liability insurance** carriers for further advice.

An example of an incident report template appears in Figure 5-1. Readers are encouraged to adapt this shell form to their own use, with permission of, and in consultation with, their own legal advisors.

QUALITY MANAGEMENT

Quality is an elusive and enigmatic concept. How do you define *quality* as it relates to physical therapy clinical patient care service delivery? This fundamental question is key to successful physical therapy clinical management.

Generically, *quality* may best be defined simply as a subjective impression by a customer or client of the relative value of a given good or service. For physical

Date, (24 Hour) Time, Location of Incident:

_____

Description of Incident and Scene:

_____

_____

_____

_____

Parties and Witnesses:

1.

2.

3.

Action(s)/Disposition:

1. Of Persons:

_____

_____

2. Of Report:

_____

_____

Additional Comments:

_____

_____

_____

_____

_____

_____

_____

_____

Drafter's Printed Name, Signature, Time, and Date

_____

FIGURE 5-1 | Example of an incident report template.

therapy, quality of care delivered is normally measured by the subjective opinions of relevant others (e.g., patients and clients, peers, competitors, accreditation entities, educators, community leaders, media personnel, vendors, and relevant others) about the level of care along an invisible visual analog scale (with indicators of high, average, and low).

Quality is directly affected by management activities carried out by clinical managers and care professionals in particular practice settings. No managerial role, except perhaps human resource management, is as critically important to practice success as **quality management**.[26]

In terms of external oversight of quality in health care service delivery, the modifiers and definitions of quality have undergone substantial evolution and fine-tuning over the past several decades. From labels of quality assurance to total quality management to continuous quality improvement to **improvement of organizational performance**, quality management is just that: quality management. No person, organization, or system can ensure quality, just as no one can ensure any other outcome. What individuals, organizations, systems, accreditation entities, governmental agencies and bodies, patients, clients, and relevant others can do, however, is purposefully intervene, monitor, and make appropriate adjustments to services and products to continuously strive toward optimal product or service delivery in commercial transactions (including health care). That is what quality management is all about.

The originators of quality improvement, known worldwide in business as *kaizen*, are the Japanese. They have recently begun on a large scale to express self-doubt about their own continued adherence to W. Edwards Deming's quality principles [43] that gave them the preeminent competitive edge in world commerce in the 1950s, '60s, and '70s. Companies such as Sony and Toyota have begun to reconsider and retool their operations to refocus on quality and the best ways to optimize it.[9]

For health care organizations and systems, the principal external accreditation bodies are the **Commission on Accreditation of Rehabilitation Facilities (CARF), the Joint Commission (TJC)** (formerly the Joint Commission on Accreditation of Healthcare Organizations [JCAHO]),[47] and the **National Committee for Quality Assurance (NCQA)**.[48] Each has a different domain of jurisdiction that is briefly described below.

The Joint Commission (TJC) is the largest of the three aforementioned private accreditation bodies. It assesses and accredits nearly 15,000 health care organizations nationwide, principally hospitals and hospital systems, home health entities, long-term care facilities, clinical laboratories, health care staffing agencies, and assisted living centers. The Joint Commission was founded in 1951 and has as one of its stated missions continuous quality improvement in health care delivery and public safety through systematic (every 3 years) and ad hoc monitoring of health care organizational performance. Its outcomes measurement system is called *ORNX*. Joint Commission accreditation standards address the panoply of patient management issues, from patient care to patient rights and ethics to information management to human resources management. The global goal of Joint

Commission compliance is performance improvement of member organizations through intensive focus on processes and outcomes of patient care service delivery.

Performance measures (formerly called *indicators*) are used to evaluate health care organizations during accreditation. Hospitals typically monitor one major measure per year, with the principal focus on patient care and safety. System-wide performance measures include such areas as medications, security, and wound care. Departments within health care organizations, such as physical therapy, also assess one or two performance measures on an ongoing basis (e.g., patient satisfaction with care delivery).

One evaluative model for performance assessment is failure mode and effect analysis (FMEA).[24] This quality management tool is a systematic procedure used to rank possible causes of product failure by industry and to implement preventive measures. As a quality improvement process, it was originally utilized by the auto industry in the 1960s. FMEA involves intensive oversight of component processes of an action with the goal of preventing product failure. Data and documentation about processes are crucial for its successful implementation. Like Deming's total quality management (TQM), FMEA is an industrial concept that has been applied, rather awkwardly, to health care service delivery. TQM is a 14-point quality improvement philosophy developed by Deming and adopted by post–World War II Japan in the 1950s to revitalize its industries.

The Commission on Accreditation of Rehabilitation Facilities (CARF),[45] or Rehabilitation Accreditation Commission, accredits adult day services, assisted living centers, and behavioral health and medical rehabilitative facilities. It was established in 1966 and is based in Tucson, Arizona. CARF accredits 38,000 rehabilitation facilities in the United States, Canada, and Europe. Its definition of quality rehabilitation includes the elements of individualized patient care, responsiveness, and teamwork.

The National Committee for Quality Assurance (NCQA)[48] evaluates and accredits managed care organizations (MCOs) and other health care systems, providing care to 69 million Americans nationwide. Its Health Plan Employer Data and Information Set (HEDIS) incorporates 60 performance measures, the data from which form MCO report cards that are available to the public. Its 2004 State of Health Care Quality found significant quality gaps in health care delivery nationwide that accounted for as many as 79,000 patient deaths annually, $9 billion in lost productivity, and $2 billion in avertable hospital cost outlays[41] NCQA was founded in 1991 and is headquartered in Washington, D.C.

Augmenting the accreditation activities of these and other private accreditation entities are local, state, and federal agency oversight bodies, which affect health care quality improvement largely by controlling public reimbursement purse strings. The largest of these of these is the federal Department of Health and Human Services' Center for Medicare and Medicaid Services (CMS). The agency's web site is www.cms.us.gov.[46]

Measures of quality that form the basis for health care organizational assessment and improvement include, but are certainly not limited to, competency assessments, occurrence screening, patient care assessments, patient satisfaction surveys, peer review activities, performance appraisals, time-and-motion studies, and utilization review.

EXERCISE 5-2

Consider the following facts. ABC Outpatient Rehabilitation Services, Inc., is an interdisciplinary outpatient physical rehabilitation center employing two physicians, three physical therapists, one occupational therapist, one occupational health nurse, and two aides. No one on staff has yet been appointed as quality management coordinator. The following incidents have occurred over the past 30 days: a patient fell from a wheelchair (the patient did not sustain injury); another patient developed a minor nosocomial infection during care; and one staff member failed to pass required basic cardiac life support training and testing. Focusing on these three specific problems (and not on particular people), develop a quality audit checklist consisting of 10 focused questions for investigation of each of these three adverse events. Additionally, propose in a brief simulated letter that the position of quality coordinator be staffed, and nominate someone from the center to fill that position (from existing or expanded staff).

Examples of a physical therapy patient satisfaction survey appear in Figures 5-2 (in English) and 5-3 (in Spanish). They may be adapted for clinical use by readers.

To our patients: Please help us to improve our services and your outcomes of care by carefully filling out this survey and returning it to the Patient Satisfaction Survey box. You need not provide your name or any personal identifiers. Thank you for your participation.

1. Please rate our PT service delivery overall: Excellent   Good   Fair   Poor

2. Comment on check-in time: _____

3. Comment on the time you waited to see your physical therapist: _____
_____

4. Rate the attitudes of our staff: Excellent   Good   Fair   Poor
   a. Receptionist
   b. Therapist
   c. Assistant(s)

Comments (optional): _____

5. If any staff were particularly helpful to you, please let us know so that we may show our appreciation to them: _____

6. In your own words, what did you learn about managing your own condition or problem from this encounter? _____
_____
_____
_____

Thanks for your cooperation and input. To discuss your care further, please call Mr. Tom Watts, PT, Clinic Manager at (717) 555-1222, or Ms. Misty Moanne, Ombudsperson, at (717) 555-1223. Have a great day!
Physical Therapy Staff and Management

FIGURE 5-2 | Example of a physical therapy patient satisfaction survey (English).

A nuestros pacientes: Por favor, ayúdanos de mejorar nuestros servicios y sus resueltos por rellenar esta encuesta, devolviéndola a la caja de Encuesta de Satisfacción de Pacientes. No tíene que incluir su nombre u otra forma de identificacíon. Gracias por su participación.

1. ¿Cómo fue nuestro servicio sobre todo?   Excelente   Bueno   Regular   Malo

2. Comente en cuánto tiempo tardó para registrarse: _____

3. Comente en el tiempo de esperar a su terapista: _____

_____

4. Cómo eran las actitudes de nuestro personal?   Excelente   Bueno   Regular   Malo
   a. Receptionista
   b. Terapista
   c. Asistente(s)

Comentario (opcional): _____

5. Si algún personal le dió servicio que le ayudó mucho, díganos por favor quien fue, para que lo agradecemos: _____

6. En sus proprias palabras, ¿qué aprendió usted de manejar su propia condición o problema con este encuentro? _____

_____
_____
_____

Gracias por su cooperación e información. Para hablar más sobre su visita, llame por favor al Señor Tomás Watts, Terapista Gerente a (717) 555-1222, o a la Señorita Misty Moanne, Representante, a (717) 555-1223. ¡Tenga un día maravilloso!
Personal y Administración de Fisioterapia

FIGURE 5-3 | Example of a physical therapy patient satisfaction survey (Spanish).

EXERCISE **5-3**

With the aid of a Spanish dictionary and bilingual collegial input, develop a one-page crutch gait instruction sheet for Spanish-speaking patients.

Spear reported on quality initiatives in health care organizations and departments and offered several important recommendations to equate quality of care standards with already high technical and professional aspirational standards. Spear focuses on what he calls "work-arounds" and how to minimize them. We have all experienced work-arounds, often referred to as redundancies, or "reinventing the wheel." Such redundancies often occur when new clinical professionals join the clinical staff and are unfamiliar with routines, customary practices, guidelines, and protocols. In many cases, protocols (such as perioperative protocols) should be in place but are not.

According to Spear, minimizing ambiguities of performance and work-arounds requires clinic-wide systematic analyses of individual and collective performance of key tasks.[39]

He recommended experimentation with simulations to practice and master quick iterative (repetitive) tasks as a means of continuous quality improvement, with collective feedback. Spear also specifically recommends increased managerial and professional focus on clinical quality improvement at four levels: (1) output (i.e., carrying out the correct procedure on the right patient); (2) responsibility (e.g., clarifying which professional does what tasks); (3) event(s) initiating intervention (i.e., what is done in cases such as potentially compensable events, such as when patient injuries occur in the clinic); and (4) enhanced targeting and rewarding of procedural competence and clinical excellence. A key initial question for staff is, what specifically impedes you from optimal quality health care delivery to patients?

EXERCISE 5-4

Individually or in small groups, list and describe remedial action for 10 redundancies or "work-arounds" in clinical physical therapy practice. Share results.

Harris described the first major change to drug labeling in 25 years by the Food and Drug Administration (FDA).[13] The new regulation applies only to new or updated drugs and to drugs approved within the past 5 years. Each new drug label will contain a box highlighting the risks and benefits of the medication, as well as any official changes to preexisting information about the drug, and a toll-free FDA contact phone number for patient (or provider) questions or issues about the drug. The new drug regulation also preempts certain health care malpractice lawsuits brought by patients against drug makers.

EXERCISE 5-5

What are physical therapists' roles and duties as clinicians and managers regarding minimization of drug administration and interaction errors?

Landro described quality improvement measures related to nosocomial infections and their prevention.[18] He reported that 2 million inpatients (one in 20 patients) contract nosocomial infections every year. These infections are responsible for one half of all major patient complications. Every year, 90,000 patients nationwide die from nosocomial infections.

What can hospitals and clinics (including physical therapy clinics) do? Landro recommended the use of disposable disinfectant cloths for cleansing patients' skin, disinfectant-releasing gloves worn by providers, and microbe-resistant bed sheets and plinth covers.

Landro also recommended that hospitals and clinics use electronic monitoring systems to track outbreaks or infections. What can patients do to minimize the likelihood of nosocomial infections? Landro suggested that they remind hospital and clinic staff members to sanitize their hands before touching them and to wipe stethoscopes and related equipment with alcohol before each use. One to three days before operative or wound care procedures, patients should also consider showering with 4% chlorhexidine soap.

Patients also share even broader responsibility for the quality of care delivery.[30] Physical therapy clinic managers should consider developing and posting a clinic Patient Statement of Rights and Responsibilities. Adherence to its principles by patients (to the maximal extent feasible) can be made part of the physical therapist–patient care contract for services. Copies of the Patient Bill of Rights and Responsibilities from Brooke Army Medical Center, San Antonio, Texas, appear in English and Spanish as Appendices C and D of this chapter. We personally thank the superlative medical clinical, administrative, and support staffs at Brooke Army Medical Center for their excellent care of military service members injured in Afghanistan, Iraq, and in trouble spots elsewhere around the world. Kudos!

PROFESSIONAL RELATIONSHIPS IN FOCUS

Rehabilitation professionals bear a particularly onerous (yet fulfilling) set of obligations to participants within the health care delivery system—patients and clients under their care; the families and significant others of patients and clients; the employing organizations within which they work; professional colleagues from their own and from complementary disciplines; business associates and product and equipment vendors; publication professionals; third-party payers; governmental officials and representatives; and accreditation professionals. They also owe responsibilities to care for themselves as professionals and human beings.

Health professional licensure and certification confer special solemn responsibilities on conferees, including the high duty to act as fiduciaries toward patients and clients served. As fiduciaries, licensed and certified health care professionals are responsible for placing their patients' and clients' best interests above those of all other persons, including those of employers and themselves. This lofty duty is strictly enforced by courts of law.

Subordinate to the special fiduciary duty owed by health professionals to patients are other important duties, including the duty of loyalty and trustworthiness owed to employing entities. This duty is most often a common law duty, fashioned and refined through court case opinions, but it exists in strong force nonetheless. It is this duty that requires health professional employees to safeguard employer confidential information, including patient and client lists, and not to expropriate their names for personal use after leaving an employer's practice. The duty of fidelity owed by an employee toward an employer similarly permits an employer to require a health professional employee contractually to refrain from disparaging the employer before third parties, including patients (the antidisparagement clause commonly found in many health professional employment contracts).

The nature of the professional relationship between health professional and patient or client is always either an implied or express contractual professional business relationship. In an express agreement (i.e., a typical business contract), the terms of the agreement are relatively clearly defined. The names of the parties, the nature and duration of the agreement, the amount of compensation paid by the patient or client and reciprocal consideration from the provider, and other tailored terms are spelled out—orally or (preferably) in writing. It is always a prudent liability risk management strategy to reduce all business contracts to writing and to employ attorneys to draft or review them (or both).

In the event that a provider-patient care contract is not in writing, there still are legally binding obligations affecting the clinical health care professional. Among these are the duty to carry out care competently (i.e., within the legal standard of care) and the duty to comply with the fiduciary legal and professional ethical duties of fidelity, truthfulness, and confidentiality owed to patients and clients. Other unstated but implied-in-law duties mandated by court decisions may also apply, depending on applicable state or federal law.

Providers should always insist that their patients and clients agree contractually to cooperate to the maximal extent feasible with prescribed examinations and interventions to the best of their best abilities. In this way, patients and clients become partners and stakeholders in their own recoveries.

Professional Liability Issues

Rehabilitation clinical professionals face formidable liability exposure incident to their professional interaction with patients and clients. After a single allegation of substandard care, a provider may face adverse legal and administrative proceedings in multiple venues. These include criminal court (People v. Doe), civil court (Patient v. Doe), administrative licensing agencies (State v. Doe), professional association judicial committees for ethical infractions, and certification entities for possible loss of board certification. Possible consequences of a finding or findings of culpability include monetary damage awards, incarceration, loss of licensure, loss of professional association affiliation, and loss of certification(s).[36]

It is because of the serious nature and consequences of a finding of liability that the best risk management measure that can be undertaken in health care clinical practice is to take all reasonable prudent preventive steps to avoid altogether any allegations by patients of substandard care or other care-related misconduct. This truism entails planning, implementation, dissemination, and ongoing revision of clinical liability risk management policies and procedures designed to protect patients and clients, health care organizations, and individual providers from harm.

> The best risk management measure that can be undertaken in health care clinical practice is to take all reasonable prudent preventive steps to avoid any and all allegations of harm to patients and clients.

BOX **5-2** ▪ **Recognized Legal Bases for Liability Imposition**

- Professional negligence, or objectively determined substandard care delivery
- Intentional care-related misconduct
- Breach of an express therapeutic promise made to a patient
- Patient injury from dangerous defectively designed or manufactured care-related products or equipment
- Patient injury from abnormally dangerous clinical care activities

---

Civil liability for physical and psychological injury incident to health care malpractice may be based on one or more of five recognized legal bases for liability imposition (Box 5-2).

Professional negligence, or substandard clinical care delivery, involves patient or client care that is objectively substandard (i.e., care that fails to comport with expected standards of practice for the defendant–health care provider's professional discipline (Box 5-3).

In a health care malpractice civil case, the plaintiff must prove the four elements of proof by a preponderance, or greater weight, of evidence to win his or her case. This same standard of proof normally also applies to administrative agency and professional association proceedings. The standard of proof in criminal cases, however, is much higher: guilt beyond a (i.e., any) reasonable doubt. This higher standard of proof in criminal cases applies because the consequences of a finding of criminal culpability are much more severe than with civil or administrative proceedings: loss of freedom (incarceration) and the lifelong stigma of a criminal conviction.

Breach of a legal duty owed to a patient, or noncompliance with minimally acceptable practice standards, in a health care malpractice civil lawsuit is normally proved through expert witness testimony on the standard of care, which focuses on whether minimally acceptable practice standards were met or not met by the defendant–health care provider. Often, expert witness testimony is in conflict in

---

BOX **5-3** ▪ **Elements of Proof for Professional Negligence**

Classic elements of proof in a professional negligence patient-initiated lawsuit:
- Proof that the defendant-provider (and/or health care organization) owed a special duty toward the plaintiff-patient to carry out care competently and within acceptable legal practice standards
- Proof that the defendant negligently failed to carry out care within such standards (breach of duty)
- Proof of resultant patient injury
- Proof of resultant losses (e.g., lost income, consequential medical and related expenses, pain and suffering; called *money damages*)

pretrial discovery (depositions) and at trial and must be compared and weighed by a judge or jury deciding a case. The standard of care may also be established or supported through introduction into evidence at trial of relevant authoritative reference texts and peer-reviewed journals (i.e., evidence-based practice) and discipline-specific or institutional clinical practice protocols and guidelines.

Although every legally competent person bears legal responsibility for his or her conduct (and rehabilitation professionals in particular toward patients pursuant to their special status), certain persons and entities also bear legal and financial responsibility for the conduct of others. This concept is called *vicarious liability*.

Employing health care organizations normally bear legal responsibility for the official conduct of their employees, acting within the scope of their employment. Thus it is a health care organization, and not its supervisory licensed health care professionals, that is vicariously liable for the official conduct of assistants and extender personnel.

Employers normally escape vicarious liability under two sets of circumstances. First, when an employee engages in unforeseeable conduct or blatantly impermissible misconduct, an employer might not be vicariously or indirectly liable for that conduct. For example, when an employee brings a knife to the clinic and stabs a patient, the employer might not be vicariously liable for that employee's misconduct (assuming that there was no known or reasonably discoverable propensity to violence on the part of the offending employee). Second, the employer is not normally vicariously liable for the conduct of contract professionals and their staffs. An exception occurs when the employer fails to undertake reasonable measures to distinguish contract from employed staff and a court imposes vicarious liability for contract staff under apparent or ostensible agency principles.

Irrespective of whether the patient injury results from employee, contract staff, consultant, or volunteer official conduct, the legal concept of corporate liability holds health care organizations liable for injuries to patients and others for what are called *nondelegable duties*, such as quality improvement and management programs, appropriate hiring and retention of staff, and facility safety, among other possible considerations.

Ordinary negligence for common, non–care-related injuries is not considered to be health care malpractice. Ordinary negligence involves injury to anyone (including patients) on premises caused by non–care-related physical hazards, such as unsecured electrical cords, wet surfaces, and sharp objects. Ordinary premises liability is insured against under general, and not professional, liability insurance policies. A payment or settlement to an injured person in an ordinary negligence claim or lawsuit is not normally reportable as health care malpractice to the National Practitioner Data Bank, which requires the reporting of malpractice payments and judgments involving licensed health care providers.

Professional Liability Insurance Issues

All clinical primary health care professionals should consider, in consultation with their legal counsel, obtaining and maintaining individual professional liability insurance to transfer the risk of monetary loss incident to health care malpractice to their insurer. Although employers always carry professional liability insurance on their health professional employees, the primary purpose of that insurance coverage is to protect employer interests. Supplemental (and often relatively inexpensive) individual professional liability insurance coverage adds an additional layer of liability risk transfer potential to a health professional's insurance portfolio. As of 2005, CNA underwrote 56,971 physical therapy professional liability insurance policies, up from 12,371 in 1993, a 460% increase.[31]

There are two principal types of health professional liability insurance: claims-made and occurrence policies. Claims-made policies generally insulate health professionals from liability for covered conduct only while a policy remains in force (i.e., during a period of employment when premium payments are being made). Occurrence policies, on the other hand, provide longer-term coverage so that even if employment is ended and a policy terminated, covered conduct that occurred during the term of the policy is protected from personal liability exposure.

In many or most cases, health care malpractice claims and lawsuits are filed months or years after the alleged injury. For that reason, occurrence coverage may be more advantageous for health professionals, albeit more costly in the short term. To achieve similar protection under claims-made policies, insured professionals must normally purchase relatively expensive tail or prior acts (postpolicy period) insurance coverage.

In any event, a health professional should discuss his or her individual situation and needs with state-licensed legal counsel before purchasing a professional liability insurance policy. Keep in mind, too, the fact that professional liability insurance normally does not (and cannot by law as a matter of social policy) pay for malicious intentional misconduct committed by health care providers, such as sexual assault or battery of a patient.

In addition to professional liability insurance for clinical professionals, physical therapy clinical managers must ensure that their practices are covered by comprehensive insurance, including general (non-care-related), premises liability, and employment practices (discrimination and sexual harassment) coverage.[21]

Principles of Liability Risk Management

Risk management really means liability risk management—that is, self-protection from personal exposure to monetary losses from a settlement or court judgment in a civil legal action. In this sense, risk management is a prophylaxis, or preventive measure.

Risk management is an integral component of an overall quality management program in any health care organization. However, unlike competency assessment, process and outcomes analyses, documentation and information management, resource utilization management, safety and security management, and infection control, liability risk management seemingly serves the interests of health professionals and organizations over those of patients and clients. Although this may be so, it does not derogate in any way from the ultimate duty owed by providers to patients and clients. In fact, the deliberate processes of risk appraisal and avoidance help to lessen the incidence of patient and client injury incident to care, indirectly serving patients' interests as well.

Risk management strategies and tactics span a continuum from mundane through sophisticated processes, and all are potentially invaluable as liability avoidance tools. At the simplest extreme, vigilance on the part of all health care workers regarding area safety and security is critically important.[15] In every health care setting, every worker should be a safety manager.

More sophisticated measures such as systematic and ad hoc equipment calibration and maintenance, fire and other evacuation drills, universal staff cardiopulmonary resuscitation and first aid certification, interpersonal communication training (with input from human resource management specialists), control of hazardous substances, and other devices are important as well.

One critically important aspect of liability risk management programs is the systematic involvement of legal counsel in in-service education processes. Attorneys' input into proposed liability risk management strategies and tactics, whether from institutional legal counsel or consulting legal advisors, may spell the difference between liability and nonliability for providers and organizations. Attorneys should also be tapped to provide review of important salient legal cases, statutes, and regulations, especially those related to sexual harassment and misconduct issues.

> In every health care setting, every worker should be a safety manager.

Future Directions in Risk Management

Liability risk management is as integral to fostering optimal quality patient care as are peer review; credentialing, privileging and competency assessment; equipment maintenance; and other more obviously patient-focused quality management processes. Although risk management seems exclusively self-centered and self-protective, it actually serves directly to optimize the quality of patient care delivered by providers in facilities by focusing attention on ambient safety and security.

Attorneys and facility risk managers are risk management consultants to health care providers and clinical managers and should be consulted regularly and systematically, as well as utilized in in-service education processes on a regularly recurring basis. Through effective risk management, optimal quality patient care and liability minimization become mutually inclusive goals of providers and health care organizations.

EXERCISE 5-6

Brainstorm and develop a top-10 list of clinical risk management measures that most help minimize liability exposure for you and your professional colleagues in your practice. Share results among colleagues or small groups.

SUMMARY

Management of health information is critically important and complex. Compliance by health care professionals and organizations with such statutes as HIPAA is representative of the duties owed. The principal purpose of patient care documentation is to communicate vital patient information to other health care professionals who have an immediate need to know the information because they are treating the patient. HIPAA does not hinder any provider's ability to carry out this formidable responsibility. Incident reporting of adverse events is similarly important and protects both patients and providers. Global quality management encompasses all measures implemented to optimize the quality of patient care delivered by providers and health care organizations. Accreditation entities include the TJC, CARF, NCQA, and state and federal quality oversight agencies and offices. Risk management, a component of quality management, focuses on preventing liability exposure. Health care malpractice liability is primarily associated with professional negligence, or substandard care delivery. Providers must consider carrying their own professional liability insurance coverage, preferably occurrence coverage, which protects them long after employment and payment of premiums lapse.

REFERENCES AND READINGS

1. Alderman E, Kennedy C: *The right to privacy*, New York, 1995, Alfred Knopf.
2. Atkinson W: Can you keep a medical secret? *HR Magazine* 46(6):60-67, 2001.
3. Bloom C: Peer, utilization and claims reviews of physical therapists, *Policy Watch* 30(4):1-2, 22, 2000.
4. Brailer DJ: Your medical history, to go, *New York Times*, Sept. 19, 2006, A23.
5. Continuing Care Risk Management, vols. 1, 2, Plymouth Meeting, Pa, 2000, ECRI.
6. DHHS issues first guidance on new patient privacy protections, *Health Lawyers News* 5(8): 14, 2001.
7. Di Lima SN, Waevers SB: *Health care facilities risk management forms, checklists & guidelines*, Gaithersburg, Md, 1998, Aspen.
8. Dobrzykowski EA: *Essential readings in rehabilitation outcomes measures: application, methodology, and technology*, Gaithersburg, Md, 1998, Aspen.
9. Fackler M: Japanese fret that quality is on the decline, *New York Times*, Sept. 21, 2006, A1.
10. Flecky K: The uncooperative patient, *Rehab Management* 14(6):20-24, 2001.
11. Furrow BR et al: *Health law*, ed 2, St. Paul, Minn, 2000, West Group.
12. Hall MA, Ellman IM: *Health care law and ethics*, St Paul, Minn, 1990, West Publishing Co.
13. Harris G: New drug label rule intended to reduce medical errors, *New York Times*, Jan. 19, 2006, A14.
14. HCFA changes name, announces new initiatives, *Rehab Management* 14(6):10, 2001.
15. IOM says that safety rules need a major overhaul, *State Health Watch* 8(5):9-10, 2001.
16. Krulish LH: In my opinion: a hundred and one uses for OASIS, *Home Health Section Quarterly Report* 35(1):10, 2000.
17. Kupchynsky RJ, Camin CS: Legal considerations in telehealth, *Texas Bar Journal* 64(1):20-31, 2001.

18. Landro L: Hospitals take stronger steps against bacteria, *Wall Street Journal*, March 8, 2006, D1.

19. Landro L: Tools that can help you keep your own accurate medical records, *Wall Street Journal*, May 26, 2000, B1.

20. Leonard B: Electronic signatures law may boost paperless HR departments, *HR Magazine* (Nov.): 40, 2000.

21. LePostollec M: Get covered: a comprehensive insurance package can protect practice owners from legal and financial risks, *Advance for Physical Therapists & PT Assistants* 12(4):11-12, 2001.

22. Lewis DK: Telehealth doesn't have to spell trouble, *Risk Advisor* 4(1):1, 2001.

23. Liebler JG: *Health information management manual*, Gaithersburg, Md, 1998, Aspen.

24. McDermott RE, Mikulak RJ, Beauregard MR: *The basics of FMEA*, London, 1996, Kraus Organization.

25. Mineham M: HIIS releases latest medical privacy regulations, *HR News* 20(2):1, 13, 2001.

26. Muir J: The quest for quality, *PT Magazine* May):50-57, 2004.

27. Murer C: Privacy packs a punch, *Rehab Management* 14(3):36-37, 2001.

28. *Pearls: risk management pearls for physical therapists*, Alexandria, Va, 1995, American Physical Therapy Association.

29. Pesavento P: Innovative information management, *Rehab Management* pp. 60-65, Feb. 2001.

30. Pettus MC: *The savvy patient: the ultimate advocate for quality health care*, Sterling, Va, 2004, Capital Books.

31. *Physical therapy claims study*, Chicago, 2006, CNA.

32. *Privacy of health information: a report on the 2001 public interest colloquium held March 2-3, 2001, Washington, DC*, Washington, DC, 2001, American Health Lawyers Association.

33. *Regulatory Advisory*, Chicago, 2001, American Hospital Association.

34. Sarudi D: Sneaks and leaks sink privacy policies, *Hospitals and Health Networks* 74(8): 40-44, 2000.

35. Scott RW: *Legal aspects of documenting patient care*, ed 3, Sudbury, Mass, 2006, Jones and Bartlett.

36. Scott RW: *Health care malpractice*, ed 2, New York, 2000, McGraw-Hill.

37. Scott RW: *Professional ethics: a guide for rehabilitation professionals*, St Louis, 1998, Mosby.

38. Spangler L: What's happening with HIPAA? *Texas Medicine* 99(3):19-20, 2003.

39. Spear SJ: Fixing health care from the inside, today, *Harvard Business Review*, 83(9): 78-91, 2005.

40. *Standards for privacy of individually identifiable health information: guidance*, Washington, DC, 2001, Department of Health and Human Services, 45 C.F.R. Parts 160, 164.

41. *State of health care quality*, Washington, DC, 2004, NCQA.

42. Technology trends: electronic signatures move us one step closer to paperless HR, *Workplace Visions* 6: 3, 2000.

43. Walton M: *The Deming management method*, New York, 1986, Perigee Books.

44. http://:www.ahla.org. Accessed Mar. 30, 2007.

45. http://:www.carf.org. Accessed Mar. 30, 2007.

46. http://:www.cma.us.gov. Accessed Mar. 30, 2007.

47. http://:www. jcaho.org. Accessed Mar. 30, 2007. [In 2007, the organization's name contracted to "The Joint Commission."]

48. http://:www.ncqa.org. Accessed Mar. 30, 2007.

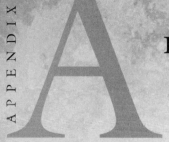
HIPAA Privacy Notification, English Version

ABC Rehabilitation Clinic
123 Main Street
Anytown, USA 65432
(333) 555-HELP

CLINIC PRIVACY POLICY

Effective date: April 16, 2003

This notice informs you of the protections we afford to your protected health information (PHI). Please read it carefully.

Purpose: HIPAA, the Health Insurance Portability and Accountability Act of 1996, is a federal law addressing privacy and the protection of protected health information (PHI). This law gives you significant new rights as to how your PHI is used. HIPAA provides for penalties for misuse of PHI. As required by HIPAA, this notice explains how we are obliged to maintain the privacy of your PHI and how we are permitted, by law, to use and communicate it.

Maintenance of records: We utilize and communicate your PHI for the following reasons: treatment, reimbursement, and administrative medical operations.

Treatment includes medical services delivered by professionals. Example: evaluation by a doctor or nurse.

Reimbursement includes activities required for reimbursement for services, including, among other things, confirming insurance coverage, sending bills and collection, and utilization review. Example: sending off a bill for services to your company for payment.

Administrative medical operations include the business of managing the clinic, including, among other things, improving the quality of services, conducting audits, and client services. Example: patient satisfaction surveys.

We also are permitted to create and distribute anonymous medical information by removing all references to PHI.

All of the employees of this clinic may see your records, as needed. We use sign-in and sign-out logs containing the names of our patients in the waiting room, and we telephone patients to confirm appointments. We place your folder in a plastic inbox (with your name hidden) in the hallway in front of your treatment room.

When making photocopies of your records, we have your folder in our sight at all times until we file it away with other folders. The medical records area is limited to employees only. When we send your PHI by fax, we ensure to the maximal extent possible that the receiving fax is secure.

All other uses of your PHI require your written authorization, including sharing your PHI with family members or others. You have the right to revoke any authorization in writing, and we have the legal duty to comply with such a revocation, except to the extent that we have used your information in reliance on your previous authorization, or as required by law.

Patients have the right to see, copy, and amend their medical records. To take advantage of this right, please present your request in writing to the clinic Privacy Officer (discussed in more detail later). You have the right to see your medical records. We will try to give you access as quickly as possible, depending on our load. Within 1 week of your request, you may see your records in one of our offices, with the assistance of one of our employees. You have the right to make copies of your records. We have the right to charge for those copies. You may also request that the Privacy Officer honor special limitations on the uses and communications of your PHI. We are not obliged to comply with such requests. If we agree, we have to comply with the request until you advise us in writing otherwise. You have the right to receive a copy of this notice, which we offer to you on your first visit. This notice, which is subject to change, is posted prominently in our waiting area.

Privacy Officer: The Privacy Officer for the clinic is _____ _____, PT, OCS. Please, speak with this employee about any question or complaint that you may have about your PHI. You may make special requests concerning your PHI.

Correspondence with the patient: We will send correspondence to the address that you have given us, but you have the right to ask that we send correspondence to a different address.

Complaints: If you feel that your PHI has not been treated with privacy, you may communicate this concern to the clinic Privacy Officer. You also have the right to communicate any problem to the Secretary of Health and Human Services (a division of the federal government) without being worried about retaliation by this clinic. We ask, though, that you first discuss and try to resolve any problem with our Privacy Officer. Thanks, and welcome to XYZ Clinic!

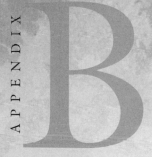
HIPAA Privacy Notification, Spanish Version

Clínica ABC de Rehabilitación
123 Main Street
Anytown, USA 65432
(333) 555-HELP

NORMA DE PRIVACIDAD DE LA CLÍNICA

Fech efectiva: April 16, 2003

ESTA NOTICIA LE INFORMA SOBRE LAS PROTECCIONES QUE TOMAMOS CON SU INFORMACIÓN MÉDICA PROTEGIDA. HAZ EL FAVOR DE LEERLO CON CUIDADO.

Intento: HIPAA, el Health Insurance Portability and Accountability Act of 1996, es una ley federal que trata con la privacidad y protección de información médica protegida (IMP). Esta ley le da a usted, el paciente, derechos nuevos significantes sobre cómo se utiliza su IMP. HIPAA provee por penas por el mal uso de IMP. Como es requisito por HIPAA, esta norma explica cómo estamos obligados a mantener la privacidad de su IMP y cómo estamos permitidos, por la ley, usar y comunicar su IMP.

Mantenimiento de los documentos: Utilizamos y comunicamos su IMP por las razones siguientes: el tratamiento, el pago y las operaciones administrativas médicas.

El tratamiento incluye servicios médicos entregados por profesionales. Ejemplo: evaluación por un médico o una enfermera.

El pago incluye actividades requeridas para el reembolso de servicios, incluyendo, entre otras cosas, confirmar los seguros, mandar facturas y coleccionarlas, y análisis de utilización. Ejemplo: mandando una factura a su compañía de seguro para pagar por servicios.

Las operaciones administrativas médicas incluyen el negocio de administrar la clínica, incluyendo, entre otras cosas, el mejoramiento de la calidad de servicios, hacer auditorías, y servicio de clientes. Ejemplo: encuestas de satisfacción.

También podemos hacer y distribuir información médica anónima por quitar todas referencias a la IMP.

Todos los empleados de esta clínica pueden ver sus documentos, si necesitan verlos. Usamos planillas de firmar al entrar y salir que contienen los nombres de nuestros pacientes en la sala de espera, y llamamos a pacientes para recordarles de sus citas. Pondremos su carpeta de documentos en un caja plástica (con nombre escondido) en el pasillo de su cuarto de tratamiento.

Al hacer copias de sus documentos, tendremos la carpeta en nuestra vista hasta que lo guardamos con las otras carpetas. La área en que guardamos las carpetas está limitada a sólo los empleados. Cuando mandamos sus documentos por fax, nos aseguramos lo más posible que el fax a donde los mandamos está seguro.

Todos los otros usos de su IMP requieren su autorización escrita, incluyendo el compartimiento de su IMP con familiares u otras personas. Tiene el derecho de revocar su autorización en escrito, y tenemos la responsabilidad de cumplir con tal revocación, excepto al punto que ya hemos usado la información dependiente de su autorización anterior, o cuando tenemos que comunicar información según la ley.

El derecho de los pacientes a ver, copiar y enmendar sus documentos médicos: Para ejecutar estos derechos, por favor presente su petición en escrito al Oficial de la Privacidad de la clínica (vea abajo). Usted tiene el derecho de ver sus documentos médicos. Trataremos de rápidamente darle acceso, dependiente en lo ocupado que estemos. Dentro de una semana después de su solicitud, podrá ver los documentos en una sala de esta oficina, con la asistencia de un empleado. Tendrá el derecho de hacer copias. Tenemos el derecho de cobrar por las copias. También puede pedir al Oficial de la Privacidad peticiones especiales sobre los usos y comunicaciones de su IMP. No tenemos que cumplir con estas peticiones. Si estamos de acuerdo, tenemos que seguir con la petición hasta que usted acuerde en escrito de quitarla. Tiene el derecho de tener una copia de esta noticia que le ofrecemos en su primera visita a la clínica. Esta noticia, que se puede cambiar, está puesta prominentemente en la sala de recepción.

Oficial de la Privacidad: El Oficial de la Privacidad de la clinica es _____ _____, PT, OCS. Por favor, hable con este empleado sobre cualquiera pregunta o queja que tenga sobre su IMP. Puede pedirle cosas en especial sobre su IMP.

Correspondencia al paciente: Mandaremos cartas a la dirección que usted nos ha dado, pero tiene el derecho de pedir que las mandemos a otra dirección.

Quejas: Si usted piensa que su IMP no ha sido tratado con privacidad, usted puede comunicar este problema al Oficial de la Privacidad de la clínica. También tiene el derecho de comunicar cualquier problema al Secretario de Health and Human Services (división del gobierno federal) sin preocupaciones de retaliación de esta clínica. Le rogamos que hable primeramente con el Oficial de la Privacidad para resolver problemas. Gracias y bienvenido a la clínica XYZ!

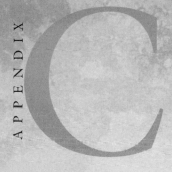

Patient Bill of Rights and Responsibilities, Brooke Army Medical Center, San Antonio, Texas, English Version

Patients' Rights and Responsibilities
Brooke Army Medical Center
Fort Sam Houston, Texas

We at Brooke Army Medical Center (BAMC) hold the welfare and safety of the patient as our highest priority. The most important person in this medical center is you, our patient. Our goal is to provide you with the best medical care available. Our success will be reflected in your satisfaction with the treatment you receive. We regard your basic human rights with great importance. You have the right to freedom of expression, to make your own decisions, and to know that your human rights will be preserved and respected. The following is a list of patient rights and responsibilities.

YOUR RIGHTS AS A PATIENT

- You have the right to receive respectful, considerate, and supportive treatment and service.
- We will do our best to provide you with compassionate and respectful care at all times.
- We will do everything possible to provide a safe hospital environment.
- We will be attentive to your specific needs and requests, understanding that they should not interfere with medical care for you or for others.
- In providing you with care, we will not discriminate on the basis of race, ethnicity, national origin, religion, gender, age, mental or physical disability, genetic information, sexual orientation, or source of payment.
- You have the right to be involved in all aspects of your care.
- We will make sure that you know which physician or care provider is primarily responsible for your care. We will explain the professional status and the role of persons who help in your care.
- We will keep you fully informed about your condition, the results of tests we perform, and the treatment you receive.

- We will clearly explain to you any treatments or procedures that we propose. We will request your written consent for procedures that carry more than minimal risk.
- We will make sure that you are part of the decision-making process in your care. When there are dilemmas or differences over care decisions, we will include you in resolving them.
- We will honor your right to refuse the care that we advise. (In some circumstances, especially for active duty patients, laws and regulations may override this right.)
- We will honor your Advance Directive or Medical Power of Attorney regarding limits to the care that you wish to receive.
- You have the right to receive timely and appropriate assessment and management of your pain.
- We will routinely ask if you are suffering pain. If you are, we will evaluate it further and help you get relief.
- You have the right to have your personal needs respected.
- We will respect the confidentiality of your personal information throughout the institution. (For those on active duty, complete confidentiality may not be possible because of requirements to report some conditions or findings.) We will respect your need for privacy in conversations, examinations, information sharing, and procedures. Also, you may request that a chaperone be present during an examination or procedure.
- We will communicate with you in a language that you understand.
- We will respect your need to feel safe and secure throughout the facility. Hospital employees will be identifiable with badges or nameplates.
- We will take your concerns and complaints seriously and will work hard to resolve them.
- We will respect your need for pastoral care and other spiritual services. Our chaplain service is on call at all times. Other spiritual support is welcome, as long as it does not interfere with patient care or hospital function.
- We will respect your need to communicate with others, both family and friends. If it is medically necessary to limit your communications with others, we will tell you and your family why.
- We will use soft fabric restraints, with close and frequent monitoring, if you become so confused that you are in danger of hurting yourself or others. We will untie the restraints as soon as we safely can do so.
- You have the right to receive information on how to contact protective services.
- At your request, we will give you information on how you may contact protective services for children, adults, or the elderly. We will do this confidentially.
- You have the right to participate in clinical research when it is appropriate.
- Your care provider will discuss this with you when it is appropriate. The Institutional Review Board, a committee that includes people from many parts of this community, monitors all research at BAMC. We will thoroughly explain the proposed research to you and ask your written permission to take part. If you choose not to take part in the research, it will not affect the care that we give you. Participation is completely voluntary.

- You have the right to speak to a BAMC patient representative regarding any aspect of your care.
- We encourage patients and families to speak directly with ward of clinic personnel if there is a problem. However, if these people cannot solve it, you may contact the patient representative at 916-2330 (clinics) or 916-2200 (inpatient tower).
- You have the right to expect that this institution will operate according to a code of ethical behavior.
- The Command at BAMC is firmly committed to managing this hospital according to the highest traditions of the military and medical professionalism and ethics. In addition, our Institutional Bioethics Committee meets regularly to review ethical topics, including organizational ethics. This committee is available to you and to our employees if a serious ethical dilemma comes up in either patient care or service.
- You have a right to receive a personal copy of these patient rights.
- Copies of these patient rights are available on any ward and in any clinic at BAMC. If you cannot locate a copy for yourself, ask ward or clinic personnel. If you have any questions or comments regarding rights, we encourage you to contact a BAMC Patient Representative at 916-2330 or 916-2200.

YOUR RESPONSIBILITES AS A PATIENT

- You are responsible for maximizing your own healthy behaviors.
- You are responsible for taking an active part in decisions about your health care.
- You are responsible for providing us with accurate and complete information about your health and your condition.
- You are responsible for showing courtesy and respect for other patients, families, hospital staff, and visitors. This includes personal and hospital property.
- You are responsible for keeping your scheduled appointments on time and for giving us advance notice if you must cancel or reschedule.
- You are responsible for providing us with you current address and means of contact (such as a home phone or cell phone).
- You are responsible for providing us with current information regarding any other health insurance coverage you have.
- You are responsible for keeping yourself informed of the coverage, options, and policies of the TRICARE plan that you subscribe to as a military beneficiary. This information is available in the TRICARE Service Office. (Beneficiary Line: 1-800-406-2832).

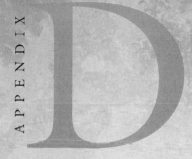

Patient Bill of Rights and Responsibilities, Brooke Army Medical Center, San Antonio, Texas, Spanish Version

Derechos y Responsabilidades de los Pacientes
Brooke Army Medical Center
Fort Sam Houston, Texas
En Brooke Army Medical Center (BAMC) consideramos que el bienestar y seguridad del paciente es nuestra mayor prioridad. La persona más importante en este centro médico es usted, nuestro paciente. Nuestro objetivo es brindarle la major atención médica disponible. Nuestro éxito se verá reflejado en su satisfacción con el tratamiento que recibe. Le damos una gran importancia a sus derechos humanos básicos. Usted tiene el derecho a la libertad de expresíon, a tomar sus propias decisiones y a saber que sus derechos humanos serán preservados y respetados. La siguiente es una lista de derechos y responsabilidades de los pacientes.

SUS DERECHOS COMO PACIENTE

- Usted tiene el derecho a recibir un tratamiento y servicio respetuoso, considerado y sustentador.
- Daremos lo mejor de nosotros para brindarle una atención respetuosa y compasiva en todo momento.
- Haremos todo lo possible para brindarle un ambiente hospitalario seguro.
- Estaremos atentos a sus necesidades y pedidos específicos, entendiendo que no deberían interferir con la atención médica para usted y los demás.
- No discriminaremos para brindarle la atención de la mejor calidad posible en función de: raza, etnia, origen nacional, religión, género, edad, incapacidad física o mental, información genética, orientación sexual o fuente de pago.
- Usted tiene el derecho a involucrarse en todos los aspectos de su atención.
- Nos aseguramos de que sepa qué médico o proveedor de atención es principalmente responsable por su atención. Explicaremos la posición profesional y el rol de las personas que ayudan en su atención.
- Lo mantendremos totalmente informado de su estado, de los resultados de exámenes que hacemos, y de el tratamiento que recise.
- Le explicaremos claramente todos los tratamientos o procedimientos que propongamos. Solicitaremos su consentimiento por escrito para los procedimientos que implican más que un riesgo minimo.

- Nos aseguraremos de que usted participe en el proceso de toma de decisiones sobre su atención. Cuando haya dilemas o diferencias en las decisiones sobre su atención, lo incluiremos a usted para resolvarlas.
- Respetaremos su derecho a rechazar la atención que aconsejamos. (En algunas circunstancias, especialmente para los pacientes en servicio activo, las leyes a reglamentos pueden anular este derecho.)
- Respetaremos su Directiva Anticipada o Poder Médico con respecto a los límites para la atención que usted desea recibir.
- Usted tiene derecho a recibir una evaluación y manejo oportuno y apropiado de su dolor.
- Le preguntaremos sistemáticamente si siente dolor. En caso afirmativo, lo evaluaremos y lo ayudaremos a obtener alivio.
- Usted tiene derecho a que se respeten sus necesidades personales.
- Respetaremos la confidencialidad de su información personal en toda la institución. (Para las personas en servicio activo, puede no ser posible mantener la confidencialidad completa, conforme a los requisitos de informar algunas condiciones y hallazgos.) Respetaremos su necesidad de privacidad en las conversaciones, estudios, información compartida y procedimientos. Asimismo, puede solicitar la presencia de un acompañante durante un estudio o procedimiento.
- Nos comunicaremos con usted en el idioma que pueda comprender.
- Respetaremos su necesidad de sentirse seguro en todas las instalaciones. Los empleados del hospital serán identificables a través de distintivos o credenciales.
- Tomaremos sus dudas y reclamos con seriedad y trabajaremos duro para solucionarlos.
- Respetaremos su necesidad de atención pastoral y otros servicios espirituales. Nuestro servicio pastoral está a su servicio a cualquier hora. Ademas, a pedido, coordinaremos otro apoyo espiritual que usted solicite siempre que no interfiera con su atención médica y la de otros pacientes o el funcionamiento del hospital.
- Respetaremos su necesidad de comunicarse con otros, tanto familiares como amigos. Si es clínicamente necesario limitar su comunicación con otros, los mantendremos a usted y a su familia informado del motivo.
- Utilizaremos dispositivos de restricción física de tela suave con su monitoreo estricto y frecuente, si usted se encuentra en un estado de confusión tal que corra peligro de lastimarse a sí misma o a otros. Quitaremos la restricción en cuanto podamos hacerlo con seguridad.
- Usted tiene derecho a recibir información sobre cómo contactar los servicios de protección.
- Si la solicita, le brindaremos información sobre cómo puede contactar los servicios de protección para niños, adultos o ancianos. Lo haremos confidencialmente.
- Usted tiene derecho a participar en investigaciones clínicas cuando sea apropiado.
- Su proveedor de atención alanizará esto cuando sea apropiado. La Junta de Revisión Institucional, un comité que incluye a personas de muchas partes de esta

comunidad, monitorea toda la investigación realizada en el BAMC. Le explicaremos detalladamente la investigación propuesta y solicitaremos su autorización escrita para participar. Si decide no participar en la investigación, esto no afectará la atención que le brindamos. La participación es completamente voluntaria.

- Usted tiene el derecho a hablar con un Representante de Pacientes de BAMC con respecto a cualquier aspecto de su atención.
- Alentamos a los pacientes y sus familias a hablar directamente con el personal clínica o de guardia si hay un problema. No obstante, si estas personas no pueden resolverlo, puede comunicarse con el Representante de Pacientes al 916-2330 (clínica) o al 916-2200 (torre de pacientes internos).
- Usted tiene el derecho a esperar que esta institución funcione conforme a un código de comportamiento ético.
- BAMC está firmemente comprometido a manejar este hospital conforme a las más elevadas tradiciones de profesionalismo y ética militar y médica. Ademas, nuestro Comité de Bioética Institucional se reune con regularidad para revisar temas éticos, incluyendo la ética organizacional. Este comité está a su disposición y la de nuestros empleados si surge un dilema ético serio en la atención o los servicios de cualquier paciente.
- Usted tiene derecho a recibir una copia personal de estos derechos de los pacientes.
- Las copias de estos derechos y responsabilidades de los pacientes están disponibles en todas las guardias y clínicas de BAMC. Si no puede encontrar una copia, solicítela al personal de guardia o de clínicas. Si tiene alguna pregunta o comentario con respecto a los derechos o responsabilidades de los pacientes, lo alentamos a que se comunique con un Representante de Pacientes de BAMC al 916-2330 (clínica) o al 916-2200.

SUS RESPONSABILIDADES COMO PACIENTE

- Usted es responsable de maximizar sus propios comportamientos saludables.
- Usted es responsable de tomar parte activa en las decisiones sobre la atención de su salud.
- Usted es responsable de brindarnos información precisa y completa sobre su salud y su estado.
- Usted es responsable de mostrar cortesía y respeto hacia los otros pacientes, familias, personal del hospital y visitantes. Esto incluye los bienes personales y los del hospital.
- Usted es responsable de ser punctual para sus citas programadas y de avisarnos con anticipación si debe cancelar o reprogramar una cita.
- Usted es responsable de brindarnos su domicilio actual y los médicos de contacto (tales como teléfono particular o celular).
- Usted es responsable de brindarnos información actual sobre cualquier otra cobertura de seguro de salud que posea.

- Usted es responsable de mantenerse informado de la cobertura, opciones y políticas del plan TRICARE a que usted suscribe como beneficiario militar. Esta información se encuentra disponible en la Oficina de Servicios de TRICARE (Línea para beneficiarios: 1-800-406-2832).

Epilogue

It is evident from the comprehensive range of variegated responsibilities presented in this book that physical therapy clinical services management is complex and time- and energy-intensive. Hopefully, the material in the chapters and the related cases, exercises, and questions have given you the basic tools you need to start or, if you are already a manager, to continue forward.

In a *New York Times Prospects* article titled "Making Health Care the Engine That Drives the Economy" (Aug. 22, 2006, D5), Kolata aptly pointed out that by 2030, 25% of the gross domestic product will be spent on health care. He equated health care to the railroads of the nineteenth and early twentieth centuries—the driving force behind prosperity and individual well-being. As clinical managers, you are in the cockpit, controlling the speed and fuel expenditure of this economic engine. It is up to you to be not only astute clinical managers but also innovative, politically proactive, creative, and inventive, so that the power of health care service delivery will not overwhelm the rest of the economy.

In a May 2006 *Harvard Business Review* article titled "Why Innovation in Health Care Is So Hard" (May 2006, 58-66), Herlinger argued that health care desperately requires an infusion of creativity in order to thrive. She encouraged clinical managers to become more inclusive of professionals from diverse disciplines and to work to halt destructive turf wars that cripple progress and unity. As physical therapy clinical services managers, you already know how to orchestrate and synthesize the efforts of diverse primary and support professionals in support of optimal patient outcomes. You must continue to bring diverse clinicians together for the common good of patients and society.

Your role as health care clinical manager is most important and your efforts are most appreciated. Again, best wishes for continuing success in all that you do to serve patients under your care!

Index

All page numbers followed by f indicate figures; by t indicate tables; and by b indicate boxes.